Don't Forget
THE Siblings

Growing up on the Sidelines of Duchenne Muscular Dystrophy

Misty VanderWeele presents:

20 real-life stories about siblings growing up knowing their brother or sister will most likely die from Duchenne Muscular Dystrophy.

Don't Forget the Siblings, Growing up on the Sidelines of Duchenne Muscular Dystrophy

2013 Misty VanderWeele (MV International)

ISBN: **978-0-9893247-0-0**

Publisher, Misty VanderWeele (MV International)
PO Box 4124
Palmer, Alaska 99645

Cover design by Misty VanderWeele

Cover and Letter from the Editor photography: Lori Safford and Kids by Kathy Mangum Photography
www.kmangumpphotography.smugmug.com

Acknowledgements

To my beloved son Luke. Thank you for giving me your trust, faith and friendship during the writing of this book. Ultimately thank you for coming into my life and giving me the most life affirming 21 years a mother could ever ask for. Your passing delayed the publishing but HAS magnified my Duchenne story telling global mission. Your continued support from the "other side" is deeply felt.

To Glen, and Jenna, thank you for standing by me, even in your personal grief of losing our Luke to provide me with the support I need so I can continue to help others touched by Duchenne Muscular Dystrophy.

To all Duchenne siblings who grow up with the knowledge that their brother or sister has an incurable, life-threatening disease. Thank you for your love, strength and courage. I am grateful for the role you play in our families. YOU HELP COMPLETE US.

To everyone who submitted a story for this book, thank you for taking the time to share how Duchenne has touched your lives and impacted your families. Without you this book wouldn't be possible.

A HUGE thank you goes out to my friend, associate and editor, Lori Safford who so willingly took on this book project at a time when her plate was already more than full.

To Jill Anne Castle, thank you for believing in this project. Thank you for helping bring the message of our Duchenne Siblings to the world. *They must always be remembered!*

To all the previous co-authors of *Saving Our Sons One Story at a Time and Saving Our Sons & Daughters II*, for paving the way for this very important book about the siblings who sacrifice, worry and love unconditionally.

Thank you to all of the Duchenne and Muscular Dystrophy organizations around the world who work tirelessly in the fight against muscle disease. Without your continued efforts, our message would not be lifted high around the world.

And finally thanks to you, the reader of *Don't Forget the Siblings,* for taking an interest in remembering the Duchenne Siblings.

Dedication

To all Duchenne Siblings around the world for the special and supportive role they play within our families.

"Remember the siblings because they are -key to making our families function with some sense of normalcy"
~Suzan Norton

What is a Duchenne Sibling?

Duchenne Siblings are the brothers and sisters who are members of a DMD family but who do not have Duchenne Muscular Dystrophy. These siblings can also be step-brothers or sisters, or half brothers or sisters as well. Duchenne is the most common "incurable" childhood muscular dystrophy. Duchenne is what they call a muscle wasting disease. Although there are many different explanations for Duchenne that vary slightly, I am going to give it to you in layman terms.

Almost all Duchenne children (mostly males) are born seemingly healthy, but as they age to about 2-4, noticeable weakness starts to appear leaving parents wondering why their children can't keep up with their peers or why they are falling all the time. Another indicator that something just isn't right is the unique way in which Duchenne children get up from the floor. They sort of spread their feet making a triangle at the knees and then slowly walk their hands up their legs until they are standing. This is known as the *Gowers Maneuver*. Doctors, usually a neurologist or orthopedist, but on rare occasions, a pediatrician, is usually able to diagnosis a child with Duchenne at this time.

Eventually school-aged Duchenne children get too weak to walk. Somewhere around the age of 10-14 is when they usually transition into a wheelchair to get around. As puberty hits muscle wasting seems to proceed on the fast track and attacks the upper body, heart and breathing muscles. Although some will die in their teens, advances in science and care treatment options have changed this statistic, allowing young adults with Duchenne to live into their twenties and beyond. Sadly however, two DMD patients a day die from complications of the disease.

Foreword

The lives of Duchenne families are consumed with the daily needs and care of the affected child or children (because DMD is genetic, many families have two or more children with the disease). The care of these children ultimately affects every member of the immediate and extended family. The pressure on these parents and siblings is overwhelming, especially as the disease progresses and the Duchenne child ages. It taxes the emotional well-being of everyone concerned. However the impact on siblings is even greater since they are the ones who not only help care for their sibling, but also worry about the well-being of their parents. These siblings have no choice but to witness the slow devastation of Duchenne on their entire family. They grow up knowing that their sibling will die from complications during or after the teen years. The Duchenne Sibling always knows that the needs of the Duchenne child have to come first. There is just no way around the fact that these typical siblings are often overlooked or sadly, sometimes even forgotten. The financial stress of caring for a DMD child and the high rate of divorce and remarriage in families with special needs children just exasperates this situation even further.

The bottom line is that we must consider the physical, spiritual, social and emotional needs of Duchenne siblings. They will experience trials in their young lives that most adults will never have to endure and they will most likely outlive their sibling(s) as well as their parents. In some families, there may only be one Duchenne Sibling (DS) who will be left alone after all of his or her family members pass away. From all of this we know that these siblings are most likely to play a special role in the life of the child with Duchenne longer than anyone else. For this very reason Duchenne siblings should get just as much support, attention and guidance as the child with Duchenne. Just like the Duchenne child has "special needs" in every aspect of their lives, DS have special and unique needs of their own. And for Duchenne parents who are overwhelmed with the needs of their affected child(ren), it is almost impossible to meet the needs of their other unaffected child(ren).

Duchenne siblings often experience a huge amount of grief and guilt, not to mention worry, frustration, anger, and sometimes even embarrassment because they are so different from their friends. Feelings of sadness, confusion and worry about what to expect and what is expected of them can overwhelm a young person. They might even have feelings of jealousy and then experience guilt because of them. Duchenne siblings sometimes even feel like they somehow caused Duchenne because they had angry thoughts or because they wished ill things to happen to their sibling. Denying or minimizing of their feelings often results. And the last thing they want is to cause even more heartache for their parents. Depending upon personality and age some DS will put the life of the Duchenne child before their own. They usually experience a great amount of fear of losing their sibling as well. The issues these children have to deal with run so much deeper than fighting over the front seat or the last cookie. More than sharing and showing each other love or simply lending a helping hand. A Duchenne sibling grows up still having to get their homework done and do their chores while wanting to have an identity of their very own without feeling guilty that they have an independence that their brother(s) will never have.

While having Duchenne in the family presents many challenges, it also provides family members with rich opportunities that are just not available to members of typical families. You will read about these opportunities and experience the deep level of maturity and compassion in the 20 stories you'll find within the pages of *Don't Forget the Siblings*. You'll also learn about the supportive role siblings play within their families and how having Duchenne in a family builds character traits like:

- Patience, kindness and supportiveness
- Acceptance of differences in others
- Compassion, care and helpfulness
- Empathy towards others and insight into coping with challenges
- Assertiveness, dependability and loyalty that come from standing up for the child with Duchenne

Having a Duchenne sibling of my own, I have seen my daughter both struggle and excel. Duchenne has molded her into an extremely compassionate and aware young lady. I provide you with a sneak peak of her journey at the end of this book by sharing a chapter of another book I am writing for her entitled *Heart Shaped Rocks*.

Another thing that makes this book special and unique is that the sibling's journey with Duchenne is being honored with each story, while lifelong Duchenne awareness is being created at the very same time.

Further the stories within *Don't Forget the Siblings* will provide you with a unique look into the lives of families with Duchenne. Thank you for taking the time to enter into our world.

Contents

Preface

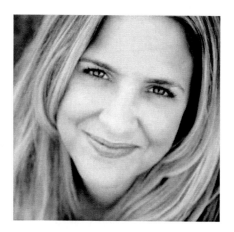

By Jill Anne Castle

I believe we are all connected. I believe in a family unit it is impossible to look at wellness unless you look at the function of the unit as a whole *because* we are all connected. Educational guru Rick Lavoie refers to this as "life on the waterbed". He explains when one person in the unit is affected in either a positive or negative way on any given day; ripples venture out and affect all those nearby. I have found in order to function in a family where one person has a chronic, potentially life limiting disorder which requires extraordinary care; it is completely short-sighted to look only at that individual. I also believe you are not doing all you can for that individual unless you take into consideration all the moving parts including yourself, your partner (or lack thereof), and the siblings.

My awareness of the sibling's role began in 2006 when I attended a workshop by Don Myer. At the time, I worked for the state's Parent Training and Information center and chose this class as one of my professional development options. I didn't know what the course entailed or what Sibshops were, but I wanted to learn.

I had no idea how it was about to change the way I parented as well as the way I viewed Duchenne Muscular Dystrophy. Up until that day, I saw Anthony, my son with DMD as the victim and my other son, Oliver as the lucky one who should just be grateful for all he had. Being motivated by pity for my son with DMD, I unknowingly projected many negative feelings onto my unaffected son. In retrospect I realized that in order to try to rectify the unjust situation, I overcompensated with Anthony in many areas while punishing myself, my husband and my other son with scarcity. Those core beliefs permeated many of my decisions in those early years.

Don Myer's non-profit organization called "The Sibling Support Project" challenged me to see a bigger picture. The first thing we learned was that Siblings have the right to their own lives and the whole family is healthier when that happens. The research showed Siblings worried about their brother far earlier than any of us expected. It challenged us to think about how we need to consider the relationship between the siblings and their special needs brother. It is most likely going to be the longest and most significant relationship in your son's life. I learned brothers and sisters want to be involved in the decisions and information in the same way we are asking them to be involved in the care. And at the end of the day, they are typical youths who have typical concerns in addition to the concerns for their brother's future.

After my training, I began running Sibshops in our area and later went on to put together Sibling panels in which I allowed the brothers and sisters to share their experiences. I have learned so much from them and still continue to learn something profoundly important every time I moderate one. I always ask the same three questions: what's good about being a brother or a sister of a child with Duchenne, what's not-so-good, and what is one thing they want everyone to know? You wouldn't believe the moving things we hear. I will never forget a young lady who chocked back the tears and said "because my parents think my brother's life may be shorter, they act as if all the important things about my life can wait because I have all the time in world". Another sibling expressed frustration with how he's not included in health discussions and decisions yet he is the one going to bat for his brother on the bus and playground. Many have specifically asked us to stop trying to protect them, because they already know WAY more than we think they do. And I always hear a lot about our expectations as parents. One kid evoked a room full of laughter by sharing that he knows his younger brother can do more for himself than his parents think because every time they leave, he "makes" him.

Then they always talk about the love. I often hear how in no way they feel their brothers are a burden. Although sometimes they wish they didn't have to skip activities just because their brother can't do them, overall it's more important to be there to support and help. Ultimately, they don't do it because they have to; they take ownership because he is *their* brother. I have found these kids to have great gifts of empathy, insight and compassion, especially for their young ages. I have also had my own son with DMD express his feelings of being a burden when the rest of us are sacrificing our own happiness. He asks to be treated normally as much as possible and that means typical experiences of his brother getting more attention as well.

For me, achieving that balance more often than not is the ultimate goal. Letting the brothers and sisters have their own lives, their own friends and their own typical experiences is key. However, respecting the right to their own lives while still not completely leaving them out of the care for their brother can be an on-going challenge. I've come to understand "fair" doesn't mean everyone gets the same, "fair" means everyone gets what they need. And everyone doesn't need the same thing. When I'm able to stop worrying about, explaining and justifying equity amongst my kids, I begin to see them as moving parts to a whole. I try my best to remember to stand back and look at how it's all working and what *all* of us need to be contributing, happy members of that whole rather than over focusing on keeping things even. They aren't.

Through my training, I also became aware of how dysfunctional some of my own expectations of Anthony's brother Oliver, really were. I made changes at home which included having occasional separate "date" nights for each of the boys, explaining that expectations for each child were going to be different because they had different needs. I began encouraging Oliver to go do more things with his friends. I wanted to make sure he knew it wasn't his responsibility to be Anthony's buddy and he didn't need to feel guilty for being able to do things Anthony couldn't. I began to set up more support for Anthony so he too could enjoy some autonomy and independence. Today, they both have their own lives. They enjoy different friends and interests while still choosing to spend time together. There are still many challenges and I believe there always will be. It's about progress not perfection.

I'm not a big fan of "everything happens for a reason". However, as I continue to watch Anthony's brother Oliver continue to grow into this incredibly special young man, I do have to acknowledge the role DMD plays in this evolution. Perhaps this isn't *why* Duchenne is in our lives, but one can certainly see the obvious gifts he is going to contribute to this world, either in spite of, or possibly even because of, DMD.

~Jill Anne Castle

Jill Anne Castle has a master in Education Psychology and a certification in Positive Behavior Support from Northern AZ University. She currently works for the Arizona Department of Education helping parents and schools navigate the Special Education process. She is also a certified SibShop facilitator, who writes, blogs and consults for Parent Project Muscular Dystrophy and MDA. She is raising two boys, Anthony, 13 and Oliver, 11 in Scottsdale, AZ.

The Millionaire's Family

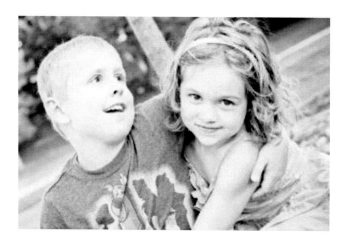

By Cindy Studlack

Cindy Studlack is a two time Duchenne co-author and mother of a son who has a Duchenne diagnosis. She lives in Minersville, PA with her family. She has also joined the fight with Misty VanderWeele and other strong parents to advocate for our children living with Duchenne. Cindy works full-time as a speech-language pathologist who assists school teams in exploring assistive technology options for elementary and secondary age students. In her spare time she enjoys running and spending time with John, her husband of 10 years, her son Colin, daughter Sara, and cat Halloween. You can contact Cindy at cstudlack@gmail.com

The Millionaire's Family

Right after our daughter Sara was born we received a comment from a sweet gentleman we did not know. He admired us and said, "You have the millionaire's family...a boy and a girl! Now all you need is a minivan and a dog!"

One year after this statement, this millionaire's family heard devastating news; "Your son has Duchenne Muscular

Dystrophy." Sara was 1 at that time and Colin was a few weeks shy of his 5th birthday. I thought, "Hmmph....some millionaire's family we are!" *In Saving Our Sons & Daughters II*, I shared our beginnings with Duchenne. The purpose of this story is to share how our life has changed as a result and how our daughter Sara helps to enrich our lives.

Fast forward to present day 2012, Sara is now 4 and Colin is soon to be 8. Colin is still walking and uses a stroller on trips that require lots of walking. Gross-motor wise Colin appears to be doing better than expected. However, there are difficulties with motor planning, limitations in social skill understanding, issues with focusing his attention, and struggles with controlling his emotions. There is not one area of Colin's life that is not affected by Duchenne. You see, DMD isn't just attacking his body; it is also targeting his ability to plan and coordinate his body movements, his ability to make and maintain friendships, his ability to learn new academic skills, and his ability to manage his emotions which often leads to frequent tantrums.

Parenting a high intensity childlike Colin is challenging at best. We are working with terrific professionals who are training our family so that we know how to manage Colin's behavior issues and help him learn. But I have to acknowledge just how much more difficult this is making our lives. Colin's sister, Sara, is a typically developing child with a strong personality. She knows her mind and is not afraid to share what she does and does not like.

Right from the beginning Sara was right in the game and not on the sidelines. As if we had a choice. Sara is determined to be right there sharing in Colin's experiences. We do a delicate balancing act giving Sara the attention she desires while taking care of Colin's needs and providing him the attention he desires. She was so happy when Colin outgrew his night splints because she has her "own" pair now. She would like it if they were pink or purple though! When we do his stretches, she lies down next to him and says, "Do mine too!" Colin's neurologist is also Sara's doctor according to her. No matter what Colin experiences, Sara also is experiencing those same things.. One day I was dropping Sara off at daycare. Her teacher stopped me to share another funny Sara story. I'm thinking, "Oh no! What did she say this time?" Sara's teacher said during morning sharing time the day before, Sara stood up and said, "I am getting a service dog! He will get my shoes for me".

In thinking about what I could share in my story for this book, I decided to offer a few laughs to the readers. These are our top 3 favorite Sara moments that we and our family and friends have enjoyed.

#3: Play versus School: On a typical school day Sara walked into the room wearing a tutu. I mentioned that she is not getting ready for play but school. Putting her hand on her hip with much emphasis said, "Well I PLAY at daycare, Mom!"

#2: Lime Green Pants Incident: On another day when Sara was 3, I went clothes shopping for Sara without her. And as you can probably guess, that was my first mistake. Mistake number two was thinking Sara would like lime green leggings to go with her pink skirt. I proudly showed her my purchases and she gave me this *mom you have no clue* look and said, "Green is NOT my color."

#1 The Lady Gaga Story:
On another day during day care, the teachers asked the kids what they did over the weekend. Most of the kids were saying the typical garden variety stuff like "I saw my grandma" or "I went to the playground". Not our Sara! She had just begun to develop a love for Lady Gaga at the time. The song *Hair* is one of her favorites. The episode went a little something like this: Sara pipes up and says "I saw Lady Gaga." Her teacher, surprised and amused, said, "You did! What did she say to you?" Sara, not one to back down said, "Well she sang a song!" Her teacher, keeping

a straight face, kept on asking, "What did she sing?" Sara, in her best singing voice, sang, "Oooo oooo oooo, I wear shark hair!" To hear Sara tell it, she encountered Lady Gaga at the local grocery store in our hometown.

Sometimes I wonder where Sara's dry humor comes from. My Dad will tell you she is me. Sara's Daddy, my husband John, is very good at quick wit and dry humor. I think I'm better at the dry humor! But seriously, I question whether it is genetics OR our life circumstance. However, I have found it to be a combination of both. I have to laugh because when she acts her 4 year old age, I usually do a double take. I typically say she is choosing to be 4 at the moment. It's funny because of her language skills and confidence you tend to forget she is as young as she is.

A friend said to me that as a family we will have deeper, more meaningful life experiences because of Duchenne Muscular Dystrophy. Sara will have a more mature outlook on life and will be stronger because of it. If Sara does not make the sports team, we will teach her to practice harder and try again. If a friend is mean to her, we will teach her to persevere and focus on better friends. None of life's challenges will keep her, or us, down for long. Because it's all just small stuff really.

One important thing John and I have learned is that Sara needs time and space to explore her own interests. She just started taking dance class and she loves it. Watching her excitement is thrilling for us. She also began swimming lessons over the summer and she recently graduated to the preschool Level 3 class! Being mindful of her interests provides her an outlet for the emotions she experiences living with a brother with special needs.

So, this Millionaire's Family will get that minivan and dog. Our dog will be a specially trained service dog and our minivan will be equipped so it is accessible for a child with mobility needs. Wherever life leads us on this Duchenne Journey, we will be prepared but will also enjoy the beauty of our unique family.

My Baby Brother is my Best Friend

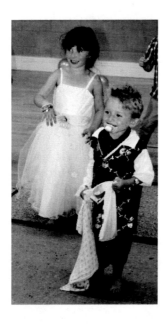

By Draven, Josie-Lee and Family

My name is Paula. I am a wife, mother and grandma. I have been working as a caregiver for 29 years. Two of my grandchildren are Josie-Lee and Draven. As their grandparent, I have been there for my daughter Jemma, her husband Jason, and the children from the start. My daughter Erica (Auntie Erica to Josie-Lee and Draven) who is a student has helped me write this story. I praise her a lot, as this has been incredibly difficult for both of us to write; but this means so much to us for Josie-Lee and Draven. All of the upsets we have faced, and everything we have been through, has brought us closer together as a family. In happiness and in sadness, we are stronger. We just want Josie-Lee and Draven to know that we love and cherish them so much. -Josie-Lee, 5 years old. Draven, 2½ years old.

My Baby Brother is my Best Friend

We (Josie-Lee and Draven's Grandma and Auntie Erica) are writing this story on behalf of Josie-Lee and Draven's Mummy and Daddy as well as on behalf of the children themselves. The purpose of this story is to share Josie-Lee's experience with her baby brother's life so far.

On the 11th of July, 2010, Josie-Lee set off for a pretty routine trip to London, though this day was different. Over the past 6 months, trips to London had been very regular for three year old Josie-Lee. She would make the hour drive to London so Mummy and Daddy could visit her baby brother, Draven, in the hospital while Grandma and Josie would go to the park or the town center. Draven spent his first seven and a half months in the Neonatal Intensive Care Unit in Lewisham hospital because he was born with TOF's (Trachea Oesophageal Fistula). This is a condition that resulted in Draven being born without his esophagus being joined to his stomach. This made it impossible for him to swallow food or drink. To fix this problem Draven had his stomach pulled up into his throat.

During Draven's stay in the neonatal ICU his only visitors were his Mummy and Daddy due to the hospital's policy. This broke Josie-Lee's heart. She wanted nothing more than to meet her new baby brother, and she did not understand why she was not allowed to see him. She only knew that Draven was sick and the hospital was helping her baby brother get better. But this trip was different. Mummy and Daddy kept telling Josie-Lee that she was going to meet her baby brother, Draven, today. Josie-Lee was beyond excited! When Josie entered Draven's hospital room the love was evident immediately. As she peered over Draven's cot, Josie's face lit up and they bonded straight away; the little family felt complete.

A month and a half later Draven was well enough to come home. This was both exciting and difficult for Josie-Lee. She was so excited to finally have Draven home, but she had to adjust to not being the only child at home any more as well as having lots of home visits from doctors and nurses. It was a very big transition for Josie, but she and Draven began to build a stronger sibling bond and it felt like the worst was over and the family could move forward with happiness.

In May of 2011 we received the devastating test results and the diagnosis of Draven's Duchenne Muscular Dystrophy. This was absolutely heart breaking for the whole family. We tried our best not to show our emotions around Josie-Lee and Draven, But Josie-Lee is a very smart little girl and she often found it easy to pick up vibes from us. Children can sense when something is wrong. Draven's needs became more demanding with more frequent trips to the London hospital, and Josie-Lee was very emotional because quality family time was affected, even though Mummy and Daddy gave Josie lots of love and affection.

Things worsened for Josie-Lee in September of 2011 when she started school a week and a half after her fourth birthday, her emotions overwhelmed her and being too young to understand why, she often expressed anger by throwing tantrums (crying and screaming) throughout her school day. Josie-Lee's teachers are aware of the family's circumstances and have helped Josie-Lee learn to manage her feelings through counseling. The school's support has benefitted Josie-Lee's attitude a great deal.

The first few months of this year were difficult. Draven broke his legs twice in the space of four months. The breaks were spiral fractures which Draven had received from simply falling over. Due to Draven having "uncommon" spiral fractures, the hospital thought it best to get the police and social services involved because they believed abuse had taken place in the home. It was horrific for us to be accused of harming our baby boy. After demanding blood tests, the authorities were told that Draven's iron and vitamin D levels were incredibly low, causing his bones to be very fragile. This explained the spiral fractures.

With Draven's first spiral fracture, he had to stay in the hospital for three weeks in traction. This upset Josie-Lee again as she doesn't like to be away from her baby brother. The bond that Josie-Lee and Draven have is incredibly strong now; they love each other to bits and are like two peas in a pod. There is nothing better than hearing these two giggling together. Josie-Lee is very protective of her baby brother, she is forever helping him. She has developed into a little Mummy and it is very adorable to watch.

It is very hard to say when will be the right time to explain Draven's DMD to Josie-Lee, only time will tell. DMD is not easy to hide. As Draven gets older, the signs of DMD show more, and Josie-Lee is starting to notice them. They are both aware that there is something happening, they just don't know what. Draven is only two and a half; we are all dreading the day when they both know about DMD and how it is going to affect each one of them.

But until the right time comes, we will make sure that we bring nothing but happiness and love to both Josie-Lee and Draven. We want to give them the best memories together and to let nothing take away their beautiful smiles.

We will NEVER stop fighting for a cure for Draven and everybody who is fighting this disease.

Best wishes and love to all,
Draven, Josie-Lee and Family

James and Jacob Daniels

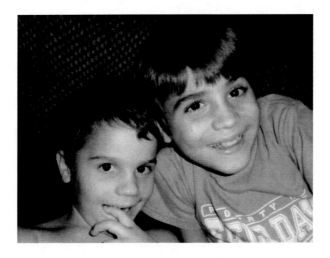

By Sarai Daniels, sister of James and Jacob (age 12)

The Race

It came from the start, without us knowing, that broke our hearts, and their bodies kept on slowing.

Two boys with hearts as long as a pole, just keep on racing, and that is their goal.

Not stopping without a prayer and never looking back, where no one is there, but always looking up, ready to be packed.

When they cross the finish line, they will be greeted by a bigger family, and certainly will shine, that's where they will be, thankfully.

And then they will walk in peacefulness and joy and their hearts never will be destroyed.

My Brothers James and Jacob: By Tabitha Daniels (age 8)

James and Jacob are my brothers. They are very nice and I love playing with them. James and I are pals. We always play with each other. Even though James is older than I, I still take care of him, but he gets mad at me when I do. When I tell Jacob not to go somewhere, he might scream, but he doesn't mean to be bad. Sometimes people in our school make fun of them and I don't like it. Jacob doesn't talk, but he's smart, so don't laugh at him. James is slow, but you shouldn't make fun of him and call him a slow poke because that is mean. If you see James or Jacob fall, then you should ask, "Are you ok?" Then help them up. I love my brothers and you should, too!

The Love of a Brother

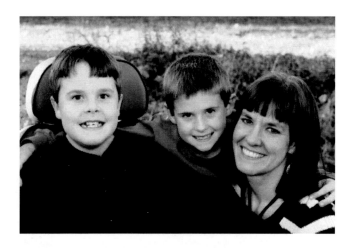

By Debra Canter

Debra Canter resides in Ozark, Missouri, with her husband and two boys. Her oldest son was diagnosed in September of 2007 with Duchenne Muscular Dystrophy when he was 5 years old. .Debra's story in Don't Forget the Siblings is her first published work. She is proud to tell the story of her two boys and how Duchenne has impacted their lives. To follow their Duchenne journey visit: www.caringbridge.org/visit/thomasjaycanter.

This story is about my two boys, Thomas and Enoch. It is a story about how their love for one another supplies the strength, courage and hope to endure life's challenges. Love is an amazing human quality. In the Bible, 1 Corinthians 13:4-7 says, "Love is patient, love is kind. It does not envy, it does not boast, it is not proud. It is not rude, it is not self-seeking, it is not easily angered, it keeps no record of wrongs. Love does not delight in evil but rejoices with the truth. It always protects, always trusts, always hopes, always perseveres." These Bible verses really convey the depth and scope of love. My boys teach me every day about the meaning of love.

Thomas is my firstborn son. He was born on a cold day in January of 2002 with snow flurries drifting about outside. He loves to draw and play video games. Thomas enjoys putting Legos together and playing with Sonic and Star Wars action figures. Thomas doesn't like to draw attention to himself. He is shy, intellectual and conscientious.

Enoch is my second and last born son. He was born on a crisp autumn day in October of 2004 when the leaves were at their peak fall color. He is energetic and likes to be funny and act silly. Like his brother, he also enjoys creating with Legos and playing video games. He is tender-hearted, smart and athletic.

There is an important detail to point out. Thomas has Duchenne muscular dystrophy; Enoch does not. For those not familiar with Duchenne, here is a quick synopsis of what is happening to Thomas. His muscle cells are unable to operate properly. They are suffering progressive damage as he moves about each day and eventually his muscle cells will die and he will lose strength throughout his body. As each year passes, he requires more and more help as his condition progresses. The challenges of Duchenne give my boys daily opportunities to know love and to give love to one another.

Thomas knows love in the way his brother cares for him. Enoch will help Thomas get toothpaste on his toothbrush. Enoch takes off Thomas's leg braces when they begin to hurt. Enoch fills up Thomas's cup with fresh water at bedtime. When Thomas accidently drops a toy, Enoch picks it up. Enoch will help Thomas with his chores, like getting the table ready for a meal. When the help required is beyond his capabilities, Enoch seeks out my husband or me. Enoch gives love by helping his brother when he is in need of assistance.

Enoch knows love in how his brother thanks him and honors him with his words. Enoch sees the relief and gratitude on Thomas's face. Enoch recognizes his brother's dependence on others to take care of him. And Thomas gives love in the way he expresses his appreciation and in exhibiting patience while Enoch attends to his request.

In the way my boys show love for each other, I see how they are strengthened. Thomas is able to trust his brother, to turn to him when he is in need and know that he is cared for. Enoch is strengthened in character as he learns selflessness when he puts his brother's needs above his own.

To wake up every day to a body that doesn't work properly is unimaginably hard. The challenges Thomas must face are seemingly insurmountable. Enoch's love for his brother in the little details of helping him with toothpaste, getting him a toy, or simply playing a video game with him is a source of encouragement to Thomas. Thomas feels valued and supported and the challenges of Duchenne fade away for a time. I see how Thomas displays great courage in his dependence upon others. I am humbled by the trust he places in his brother and thankful for Enoch's willingness to serve. With his acts of kindness in helping Thomas, Enoch gives Thomas courage to embrace each day because Thomas knows his brother is there for him.

The love expressed in being kind and putting someone else's needs before your own also provides hope. Both the giver and the receiver benefit. For instance Enoch's presence, when Thomas needs his father or me, is a source of relief. Being there when he is called to serve gives Thomas hope. And Enoch as the giver gains purpose and value. Enoch sees his action bring about good. His choice to help his brother shapes his character, transforming him into a caring, compassionate person. How Enoch chooses to help his brother is beautiful to see and gives me hope. In the end, when a life is passed away, knowing you loved them will be the greatest treasure of all.

Now don't get me wrong, every day is not all wonderful and there are many times when love seems absent. The reality of life is that there are ups and downs. We are not always rested and at our best. We sometimes act selfishly. My boys bicker over toys and video games and sometimes hurtful words are said or mean actions are taken. I find myself wondering where is the love? But when the dust settles, there is sincerity of heart and apologies are made. They may need some help along the way. Help from me or their father to illuminate how the toys and video games will fade away but their love as brothers will not and must be protected. On their own, though, they show us that they understand.

Their understanding is demonstrated in the fact they want to share a room together. There were a few times over the years that the boys had separate rooms. But they kept wanting to have sleepovers in each other's rooms and it was plain to see they just wanted to be together. Enoch's presence in particular is a source of comfort for Thomas. Thomas feels safe and protected with Enoch in the room. Something else to point out is they have bunk beds. Due to Thomas's weakened body, Enoch sleeps on the top bunk. But the interesting part is that despite the fact that they are in the same room with their respective beds, they will still have sleepovers with Enoch camping out either on the floor or on a cot next to Thomas's bed. It is truly endearing and a quiet show of the love they have for each other.

They think of each other whenever they are apart. For example, when Thomas visits the dentist and gets to choose a toy from the prize drawer after his cleaning, he will always ask if he can pick a toy out for his brother as well. And when Enoch went to the bank with me the other day to cash his birthday check, he was offered a lollipop from the teller and without hesitation asked if he could get one for his brother too. These gestures show how much they care about each other.

These stories, of sharing a room and thinking of each other when apart, show that love transcends the pettiness. Their love as brothers cannot be destroyed by minor squabbles over toys or games. It is everlasting. My boys have a bond that connects them in a special, unique way. I am so grateful that we had two boys. Knowing they can lean on each other brings me joy. Seeing how they acknowledge their need for each other brings me peace. I pray that they always recognize how important the love of a brother is.

There is sadness, heartache and pain along this journey we must walk with Duchenne. We can choose to be angry. We can choose to let frustration get the better of us. But that gains us nothing but additional heartache and despair. By choosing to love despite the difficult circumstances we find ourselves in, we can rise above and experience joy and peace. Regardless of all the good, bad or indifferent, Duchenne is a part of Enoch's life just as much as it is a part of Thomas's. But the way my boys choose to love each other and the way our family chooses to love one another, gives us the strength to persevere, the courage to stay in the fight, and the hope we need to endure the journey. I pray that you will be encouraged to love despite your circumstances and live out your life with strength, courage and hope.

Siblings in Africa – Our story of Hope and Love

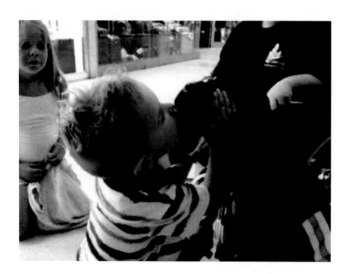

By Colin McKenzie

Colin and Suzanne McKenzie live in South Africa with their 4 children, Justin (Son of David and Suzanne), Joshua, Jessie and John. We live in a country of opportunity and many challenges resulting from the country's history, however it is home to us. We live in a country where there are many less fortunate than we are and hence we have started in our small way to change the face of Duchenne here; our site www.tmct.co.za tells the story.

Siblings in Africa – Our story of Hope and Love

Duchenne was a word the McKenzie family heard for the first time in 2006. It is a word that has changed the way we live as a family here in South Africa and it has brought us closer together. For me as a father and husband, DMD has given me the realization that life is too short to procrastinate. As a family we live one day at a time; our motto is "Make each day count".

In our story, we would like to share about the day we decided our daughter Jessie needed another sibling. Jessie has two older brothers, Joshua and Justin, who were both diagnosed with Duchenne in September 2006. Justin was 6 at the time and Joshua was 2. Our little princess was just shy of her 1st birthday.

As parents of Duchenne boys, you go through many emotional states from the time you are first told about your children's condition. You grow in many areas as a person, but for us, it was the spiritual growth that was greatest. It gave us a true understanding of the greatness of our Father. During this time, we have accepted that these boys are with us for a reason, to teach us many things about ourselves. It has also shown us who our friends really are amongst the many people we know and love.

A few years after that fateful day in 2006, we started thinking about the future. It became apparent that our little Jessie would statistically be left behind; having lost her entire family by the time she turned 30 – her parents as a result of our age and her brothers as a result of their condition. We realized how important our siblings are to us as the parents of these remarkable young boys and how blessed we are to have siblings. We knew that as we go through life, we would need more and more time to care for our sons and this might result in our little princess being left almost as an only child. It came to us that we needed to ask to be blessed with a sibling for our daughter, a sibling that would be there for her when we were occupied or no longer around, a friend and playmate.

At this time we researched the world for answers on how to proceed. When we discussed the plan, I do not believe any person we spoke to, including our families, agreed with convinced our decision to have yet another child. Imagine, we have the financial responsibility of three children already, two of whom will require significant financial support due to all the medical and other needs they will have. How could we be so irresponsible to want another child under these circumstances? It was this that caused us to doubt our faith and we "convinced" ourselves that should this child have Duchenne, we should do the right thing and terminate the pregnancy. Suzanne is a true mother and one that has always believed that God created her babies, and she was having him or her no matter what. BUT, we conformed to society and explored all the options. Of the various options, we chose the one in which when Suzanne became pregnant, we would have a CVS done at 11 weeks. Within a few weeks we would know if the baby had Duchenne and we would terminate. Simple, yet a process very strange to our way of thinking.

Throughout this time, I always believed that this sibling would be a blessing from our Father. I knew that He understood our situation and would provide us with His blessing. However, we would try to appease the people (our family and friends) and do the "right" thing.

At 11 weeks, Suzanne's gynecologist made all the arrangements to have the CVS done by a leading doctor in this field. Off we went to discover that the leading doctor had taken leave and that her partner was to do the procedure. He inserted the long needle and started to withdraw test matter when the needle separated from the syringe (was this what happened or was it a lack of skill?) and he removed the needle. In my mind, he had now conducted a procedure that had a 1:100 chance of miscarriage. He now prepared the needle and stated that he needed to re-insert it and draw more test matter. I was not happy, I knew that we were now doubling the risk of miscarriage, but we agreed to continue the procedure. As the needle was re-inserted, Suzanne had extreme pain, not present in the first incursion. The pain settled and he continued. He then withdrew the needle and was about to re insert it for a 3rd time. It was at this time I told him that he had done enough and that he had better find suitable and sufficient test matter in the samples he had already drawn to conduct the Duchenne test. I am not usually a violent person, but that day the doctor stood a great risk of being battered.

This time was extremely difficult for Suzanne and me. I often refer to it as the time I was "married to an iceberg". The anticipation of finding out whether or not our latest blessing was to be terminated just changed our moral. It also seemed that everything was against us. First the late change of the specialist to recover test matter and the complications around that process. Second, we had a call from the lab, as the doctor had forgotten to take a specific sample from Suzanne to differentiate her genetic material from the fetus. Third, we had a call from Suzanne's gynecologist, confirming that she would not be available to terminate as she would be on leave with her family, but that she had made arrangements for it to be done. Last was the issue of who would give us the results., Suzanne's psychologist was not acceptable as she is not medically trained, the gynecologist was out of town, and the genetics councilor needed her to be told by a trained professional due to the nature of the result and the consequence (as if we did not already understand this). This would mean going into the lab, a very cold and foreign place to us, which made it worse as no one we loved or who understood our family would be present with us on that defining day.

After a week we got confirmation that there were no "routine" problems identified in the basic five tests conducted and that the sex was male. It was at this time I was married to a corps. We knew that we were down to a 50% chance of losing our child. The Duchenne genetic test was then done now that we knew it was a boy. This test takes a little longer, and is only done once the sex of the baby is known.

I then researched the world for someone who had experienced a similar situation and found a family in Texas. I worked out that the mother had to have known at the time of having her 3rd child but definitely by the 4th, that Duchenne was a reality in their lives. I sent her a message asking her exactly how she managed to have 4 children, and I assumed that she had to have known about Duchenne. The answer was simple "These are God's children and they have given me as much joy and happiness as any child would. God knows and He will only give you blessings you can deal with…" It was late on a Wednesday evening here in sunny South Africa. I went to bed and spoke to my wife. I said something along the lines of "Suzanne, we are going to have this child and siblings for our children, I do not care what society thinks, until they understand our lives and our walk with God, their opinion does not count. There were loads of tears and much joy as we discussed our future family. The next morning we decided to notify all the people who had been involved in the process. Suzanne called the gynecologist to confirm the 15 week appointment on her return from leave; I called the genetics lab and suggested they send the results to whomever they deemed fit, but at least to our gynecologist as we were not interested in knowing the result for purpose of termination--we were having this child!

That Friday, I was sitting at my desk in the home office, discussing something with my younger brother at around 09h30 when I heard a screech from the bedroom. It was Suzanne, and before I could get up to investigate, she was on my lap in her night shirt overwhelmed with what was later to be determined as extreme joy. You see unbeknownst to us, our amazing gynecologist had made arrangements for the genetic councilor to call her with the results anyway while she was away. She then called Suzanne to let her know that our little man was tested and found to be non-Duchenne. Today, as I sit here and write these words, tears still come to my eyes as I remember that day.

On the 19th December 2009, early in the morning, about a week prior to the planned C-section, Suzanne's waters broke and we were off to hospital. It was a busy day at the hospital, a number of mothers expecting arrived that day, some prematurely to give birth to their children. We waited patiently as each birth was attended to. At around 12h15 we received our blessing from our Father, John Luke McKenzie. From the very minute our little Jessie learnt she had a new brother, she did not leave my side. She never missed a visit to mom and John in the hospital. I would like to believe it was because she was so happy with her new baby brother " John John baby Luke" as she called him, but it was more likely a little bit of anxiety and jealousy with the new arrival.

"John John baby Luke" is nearly 4 years old as I write this and he lives up to the meaning of his name "Blessing from God".

As a family, we would like to dedicate our story to the late Charlene de Jager, Suzanne's gynecologist through all the children's pregnancies and births. Sadly she passed away earlier this year at the tender age of 48. She was a part of our joy and sorrow, a true professional in all aspects. RIP Charlene, we miss you, till we meet again.

Defeat Is Not an Option

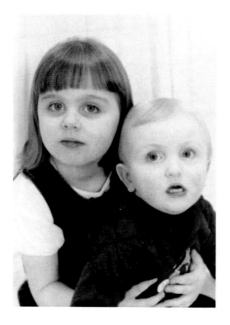

By Laura Villeneuve (Adam's Sister)

Laura Villeneuve: If you want the basics, here they are. My name is Laura Villeneuve and I am thirteen years old. I believe that sending in a story to SOSD2 is important because I will be in a book with lots of other people who may or may not be going through the same process I am. I also wanted to do this because I always tell my brother's 'story'; and I wanted people to hear my side of his story. You can contact me at: karavee@comcast.net

Defeat Is Not an Option

Let me just say right off the bat that I don't want your sympathy. My brother, Adam, is eleven (He turned 11 on 11/11/11) years old and has Duchenne Muscular Dystrophy

(DMD). My name is Laura. I'm thirteen years old, and eight years ago, my life, along with the rest of my family's lives, changed forever.

Adam was four years old when he was diagnosed with DMD. I was only six, and I don't remember much of what happened back then. All I know is that my parents were devastated and scared. I don't remember feeling scared, just confused. The first memory I have of saying or knowing anything about DMD was when I was nine and shared a news article about DMD to my fourth grade class. I understood everything the article was saying, but no one, not even my teacher, knew anything. I didn't know how that could be, but as I explained DMD, I felt warm, as if sitting by a fire. That feeling I had has stayed with me all my life, and I still love that feeling. As I look back on it now, I believe it was obvious that I was feeling that way because I was doing a good deed.

Fourth grade was one of the best years of my life, and it changed me. It was during this time that I became inspired to help my brother and others with DMD. I have worked at multiple MDA events and am an advocate for raising money for Adam and others like him, including the annual MDA walk. It's my little way of helping that makes a big difference. In a way, I'm glad that I am part of a family that lives with DMD, because now I can contribute to finding a cure to save other people's lives and that warm feeling never goes away.

A few months ago, I was on the school bus with some of my peers, and we were talking about disabled kids. The others were saying how it would be nearly impossible for a person to live a disabled life, and I greatly disagreed. I told them that my brother lives a disabled life and he is doing very well. Everyone turned to look at me, minor shock on their faces by what I said, and I was a little surprised that they had known me for so long and didn't know about Adam. I told them Adam's story, and one girl said she was sorry, but I waved her off. She had nothing to be sorry for. It wasn't her fault Adam has DMD, and I was sick and tired of sympathy and apologies. I don't need those things. The only thing I need is doctors and researchers to do their jobs and find a cure for DMD.

I told Adam's story again a few days later. I was in advisory, and my teacher asked each of us to write down something that no one knew about us. I wrote down Adam's story, and I was given the opportunity to explain DMD again, but this time I was pretty certain that, at this age, most kids would be able to understand the story better and would listen in a different way than when they were nine. A few of the people there had known me for years, and had heard Adam's story already, but others reacted the same way as they did four years ago. This didn't bug me as much, but I was still a little surprised that I had known these people for such a long time and they still didn't understand. DMD is a big part of my life, so I thought after six years they would have at least retained some of the knowledge from the other times I have talked about Adam.

I wish I could explain DMD to my entire school, but I couldn't do it with my siblings there. All three of my younger siblings are in elementary school and live with DMD as well, and I couldn't tell the story of our family on my own. Other times that I have talked about Adam and people's expressions have gone from curious to sympathetic. This drives me insane. Sympathy won't save Adam's life, so I don't need it. It brings me the opposite of comfort. People sometimes become extra careful because they are afraid that I am so upset about Adam that anything they say will make me start bawling. That is not the case at all. I have learned to live with a disabled brother.

DMD has taken an emotional toll on my life, and I have mixed feelings about it. Most days I forget about it entirely, but other times I wish I was in a different family. There was one instance a few years ago when Adam had gone into a classroom full of kids my age and they all commented to me later that they "couldn't believe how cute he was". For about a week I was only the girl with the cute little brother. This really upset me because I knew that people couldn't come to know me better if all they saw was Adam.

My life has also changed physically because of DMD. Our original house was not fit for a disabled person, much less a disabled young child. My parents decided to solve this problem by donating our house to the fire department. In 2008, the fire department burned down our house. My dad has built our new house to his specifications, meaning that it has elements that can be used by a handicapped person. This includes an elevator, a roll-in shower, and a wheelchair ramp.

Everyone is different and everyone has flaws, and Adam's is DMD. It is a big part of his life, but he is also loving, caring, respectful, funny, and sarcastic. I do worry about him though. He's in fifth grade now and from what I remember from my fifth grade year, my peers weren't that accepting of someone being different, and things that happen in fifth grade change people. The kids who bully Adam in fifth grade will continue to bully him all throughout junior high. I would hate to see Adam come home upset because people were teasing him. If he does, I think I'll need to have a talk with these kids. No one makes fun of my brother. I don't care how little you know, you should be smart enough to know that Adam is different, and he can't change.

Duchenne Muscular Dystrophy has changed my point of view on life. You only live once, and you shouldn't have to worry about a chronic disease. Adam doesn't need that. No one needs that. I can try my hardest to work toward a brighter future for Adam, but that's all I can do. I will work for him though, even if it means going to the extreme. If I was given the option to die and have all DMD patients be cured, or live and have only my brother saved, I would choose to die, because it wouldn't be right to see other families suffer and feel the guilt of only saving my brother. I would give my life to save every DMD patient, not only Adam. Defeat is not an option if someone's life is on the line, and I would rather die than surrender to Duchenne Muscular Dystrophy. I don't like thinking about what could happen if his disease becomes worse. Adam takes steroids every day to keep his muscle strength, and he has yet to be forced into a wheelchair. I think about him every day, and what could happen as he becomes older. One day my mom told me that Adam had had trouble falling asleep, and she told me it was because he was scared of the future. Kids with DMD have an increased chance of dying young, as early as the age of seventeen. Adam was scared that this was his fate. When I heard this, I wished instantly that the disease was gone and had never come near Adam or our family. I still wish for that, but since the disease is affecting Adam, the only thing I can do is try my hardest to raise money for him and pray that doctors and researchers find a cure before it's too late and the world loses another extraordinary little boy to this horrible and heartbreaking disease.

Bad News...Good Attitudes

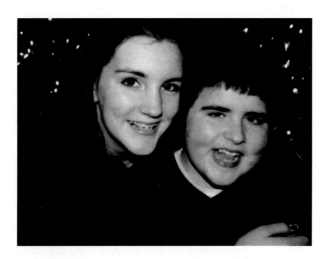

By Shannon Kearney

Shannon Margaret Kearney is 13 years old. She is in the 8th grade at South Orangetown Middle School where she is a member of the National Honor Society. She lives in Orangeburg, NY, with her parents Peter and Eileen, and her brothers Brian (15 years old) and Kevin (10 years old). She has many interests and activities that keep her busy all the time! Shannon loves to play the piano, guitar and violin. She enjoys playing basketball and volleyball. Shannon is an extremely determined young lady and a wonderful friend, sister, and daughter. She hopes to one day be a teacher like her mom.

Bad News...Good Attitudes

I've known him since the day he was born. I was young but excited about what was happening. I was getting a baby brother. When he was born I loved everything about him, and I still do. On that day, I didn't know how much that little baby in a blue blanket would change me. But this is how my baby brother, Kevin, changed my life.

For the first two years, Kevin was a normal, happy baby and I loved playing with him. But all that changed one day. The doctor called to tell us that Kevin had Duchenne Muscular Dystrophy, a muscle wasting disease. I don't remember that day clearly, but I remember my parents crying a lot. I soon learned that Kevin was going to progressively lose his muscle strength and have to be in a wheelchair when he was older. I remember that Kevin wasn't able to crawl like other babies could. He would just scoot on his behind. That was an early sign that he had DMD. I was only about 4 or 5 years old, so I didn't understand how bad this really was.

Even though Kevin has this disability, he is still a very happy kid who loves to play games and whatever sports he can. Kevin is 10 years old now and he's started to understand his weaknesses, but that doesn't stop him. My parents signed him up for a program called *Buddy Ball*. Kids with special needs each get a "buddy" each week to play sports like basketball and soccer. Kevin loves to go because it's made for kids like him. My parents try to do whatever they can to make him feel special and to allow him to do whatever the other kids can do. As he grows up, I can tell that Kevin gets upset when he sees other kids running and jumping, because he can't. I don't know how that feels, but it must tear your heart apart to constantly see people doing stuff that you can't do. But Kevin still tries his best to play and run around. When he goes out, he puts a smile on his face and plays. He is such a strong kid.

Recently, my parents got Kevin a motorized scooter that he can bring to school to use when walking becomes difficult. This has helped Kevin a lot because when he goes outside to play with his friends, he can drive around as fast as other kids can run. He feels like he can finally play with them. This makes him happy because he has never been able to keep up with the other kids, so this scooter is really helping him. I love watching Kevin drive around outside with his friends because I know he never had that feeling of being able to run when he's playing tag, but now he can, in a way. It brings a smile to my face because Kevin can finally "run" fast and he's always laughing while zooming around.

Something huge that we did for Kevin is that we modified our entire house to be handicap accessible. Before the construction Kevin's bedroom was upstairs. My parents knew that the day would be coming when Kevin wouldn't be able to get up the stairs. We had to gut our entire house, so we moved into a rental house the next town over for several months. My older brother Brian, Kevin, and I had to share a room. It was tough sharing a room with my two brothers and not having any privacy. Even though it was difficult sharing a room, I knew when our home was finished; Kevin would be able to get around easily. After 7 months in the rental house, we moved back into our "new home". Kevin's room was on the main floor and all the hallways and doorways were widened to be handicap accessible. We put in an elevator because we wanted Kevin to be able to go upstairs to the rest of the bedrooms and to go downstairs to play. We didn't want Kevin to feel like he was isolated on one level of the house. We have ramps in the front and the back of the house. The construction really made our house Kevin's home.

The remodeling of our house for Kevin changed my whole life. I had to give up my room to make space for an elevator, but I got an equally great room in return. I had to give up the home where I grew up and made memories for 10 years to make it handicap accessible. Even though I had to give it up, I know I'll make more amazing memories just knowing Kevin can live a normal life in our house.

Playing outside and physical activities aren't the only things that are hard for Kevin. He also has a learning disability. He has an extremely hard time in school, especially with taking tests. My mom is a first grade teacher, so she knows how to teach and work with young kids. My mom is very patient with him. She helps him do his homework and study for tests, but Kevin still struggles. Sometimes he freaks out at school at the teachers or at other kids. He always tries to do as little work as possible. Sometimes he gets so mad, or maybe embarrassed, that he throws things or cries because he isn't able to do the work the other kids are doing. My parents get upset and try to help him, but it's difficult. I know it isn't his fault that he has this learning disability; and I know that it affects him in every way. But it also affects me as well.

Although Kevin has hard times and troubles, he is still very smart. He has an amazing memory and he notices every little thing. Kevin doesn't miss a trick! He is the funniest kid I know. Sometimes he says things that he doesn't mean to be funny, but they are. The way he says things is often just funny or cute. He's always making my friends laugh and even people we don't know in public laugh because he has a very funny way of putting things. Laughter is very important and Kevin makes everyone feel better and he always puts a smile on everyone's face. Kevin likes to dance and sing and be the center of attention. If he didn't have this disease, I doubt that he would be as funny.

Kevin is also the sweetest person I've ever met. He's caring and loving. Kevin is extremely generous with everything. If he has candy, he always shares with me. He gives me little toys or stickers. He loves to share with everyone.

Kevin has recently become even happier since he got his companion dog, Schmoo. Schmoo and Kevin are now best friends. Schmoo is a lovable two- year old Black Labrador Retriever. He is trained and helps Kevin pick things up and gets items that Kevin can't get himself. When we went for an interview with the people who would give us the dog, Kevin said he wanted a dog that is fun to play with and gives lots of kisses. And that's what he got. Schmoo loves to give kisses to everyone, but especially to Kevin. Getting the dog really has made Kevin a happier kid overall. When I see Kevin happy and hugging Schmoo, I'm happier too.

DMD has changed Kevin. He has had to go through so much more than typical kids. He's different from everyone else. Whenever anything bad happens to him, I feel the pain as well. Sometimes he says things to me like, "Why did God have to make me have this disease?" and it makes me feel like crying, but I smile and say, "Because that's how God made you". I try to be positive around him. If I cry, he cries. He's such a good person. He's thoughtful, amazing, cute, smart and funny…and I love him so much.

Kevin would like to be a firefighter when he grows up, just like our dad, who is a captain in the New York City Fire Department. Kevin knows that because of his disability, he won't be able to be a regular firefighter, so he wants to be a dispatcher. Kevin wants to help people. He feels that fire dispatchers are just as important in saving people's lives as the firefighters. I love when people ask Kevin what he wants to be when he grows up and Kevin says a firefighter. Then he explains that a dispatcher is still a firefighter even though they don't go into the fire. He understands that his disability will affect what kind of jobs he can do, but he isn't giving up on his dream of being a firefighter just because of muscular dystrophy. This shows how much he loves to help people and how strong he is for wanting to get around his disability.

Kevin's disease affects me in many different ways. I am a different person because of Kevin. I have learned that people go through tough situations even though you can't always tell from the outside. I do get upset a lot when my parents have to help him more than me, but I'm thankful Kevin has our parents to help him. I also get upset when Kevin falls or gets hurt because I know that if he didn't have this disease, he wouldn't have to go through the pain of needing help to get up. Sometimes I feel like Kevin is more important than me because people give him more attention, but I know that he's not more important, he just needs more help.

This disease has changed Kevin into a wonderful person who understands the hardships that people go through. He's very compassionate. He's stronger than a lot of other people, especially at 10 years old. He's not physically stronger, but emotionally. He finds the good in everybody. He has turned something bad into something good. He's a ball of happiness and he doesn't take anything for granted. He's the best brother anybody could ask for.

John & Mike

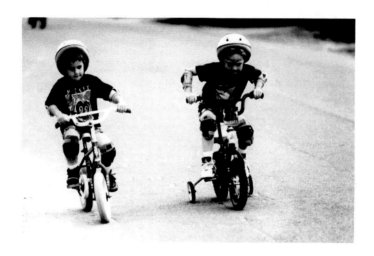

Photograph by Carl Walsh

By Suzanne Norton

Suzan Roberts Norton grew up in South Portland, Maine, the eldest of four siblings. Raised by young parents who invested their time with them, she believes that foundation has prepared her for future challenges. She is a writer, photographer, and artist as well as a wife and mother. She worked many years in the family sign business with specialties in brush lettering and calligraphy. Today she designs and hand letters ornaments, works nights at the telephone company, is a caregiver for her oldest son with Duchenne Muscular Dystrophy, and volunteers her time at a local Historical Society where she is program director and a member of the board. Occasionally she presents historic lectures for groups usually taken from stories she has written on her blog. (http://blog.likes2write.com) Physical and Mental disability awareness are causes very close to her heart. She and her husband Terry live in Maine and have two sons, Mike and John.

John & Mike

As I re-read journal entries from 21 years ago, I am shocked to read the raw emotion scribbled across the pages. I was afraid, devastated, and strong with wisdom I had not realized I possessed. Only now, when I re-read the thoughts that were in my head at the time, do I understand how wise I was for a mom of a newly diagnosed four year old boy with Duchenne Muscular Dystrophy. My world was instantly turned upside down when the doctor held my hand and told me what to expect. I was alone at Walter Reed Army Medical Center with my oldest son Mike. My husband and youngest son, John, were in Germany waiting for any news the doctors might find. I remember calling my husband at our home in Germany to share the news. I was hysterical. It must have been very difficult to hear me on the other end when he was also alone, with our other little boy.

I was worried about my son without muscular dystrophy from the very beginning as evidenced from this journal entry dated five months after diagnosis. *"I just hope in years to come, you won't feel I neglected you because of Michael. I will probably need a lot of help but as a family we will be strong. Love is everything. I have many hopes and aspirations for you. Just know that you are very important – very special. And I hope you and Michael will always be close and talk like brothers. As a family, we have a big responsibility. Michael's handicap is not only his own it belongs to all of us. And it's ok to be sad, to talk of our fears, and share in our joys. We have a lot to be thankful for- Let's always be open as a family-"*(March 18th, 1992)

I recall looking at my son, Mike, after the initial diagnosis and I felt total and utter disbelief. How could he eventually use a wheelchair? It just did not seem possible. It was almost like a terrible nightmare. After months of crying and being unable to find any happiness, I found peace through a dream one night.

Peace was a long time coming and even after 21 years, I have a newfound peace. I now realize that Mike is perfect just the way he is. I spent so much of my time fighting against Muscular Dystrophy that I lost some valuable time with him. Of course, this is my personal experience and it is different for all of us. I have enjoyed all the volunteering for nineteen years, and meeting others along the way. However, time spent with my immediate family has given me more happiness lately. I just need to enjoy our time together and focus on today.

Over the years, information I would need to share with Mike regarding his future consumed my thoughts. I was not sure how I could share this with him in years down the road. I was very careful not to share too much with anyone because I wanted to be the one to talk with him about his prognosis as he lost abilities. At times, I was premature about sharing information with him as I tried to get a feel for where he was at with what was happening with him. Once, I mentioned someone's wheelchair and maybe one day he would need the help of a wheelchair. He looked at me, puzzled, and asked if his brother would have one too. I replied perhaps not. Mike then told me that if his brother wouldn't need one, then he would not either. Another time I mentioned spinal surgery before he was ready to hear that. As parents, none of us has done everything right.

There has always been a strong bond between my two sons. From a very early age, my son without muscular dystrophy knew his brother needed assistance. He would slow down when he ran, so his brother could keep up. It was truly heartwarming to witness. As they grew to the ages of six and seven, there were some serious anger issues going on with both of them, because they did not know how to handle their emotions. We saw that they both received separate counseling sessions for a time to cope with that anger.

My son John, who was a first grader at the time, was so concerned for his brother's safety on the playground during recess, that he could not enjoy his own recess. He told me he was very worried about his brother falling and being pushed by bullies. I told him he did not have to look out for his brother, that the teachers were aware. I suppose that was easy for me to say because I was not on the playground with my brother every day. I explained to John that his brother would need a wheelchair soon. He responded by asking me why couldn't we get him one now?

In later years, through middle school and high school, they shared common friends so there was always a houseful of kids. There would be two occasions when John and Mike attended a concert and a skate park out of state. On both occasions, Mike passed out because of high $Co2$ levels. John got him to emergency rooms in both cases and advocated for his brother. One time, he was asked to leave while his brother was intubated and John refused to leave. It must have been extremely stressful for him. When a family member has DMD, the siblings also sacrifice everything and feel guilt along their journey. This weighed heavily on me over the years.

Our lives are forever changing and sometimes that change is sometimes hard to swallow. This year has been very challenging and our lives were once again turned upside in our family. We are doing the best we can by self- educating, advocacy, and showing love as well as moving forward. This is life. We have to make the best use of our time and energy. Remember the siblings because they are the key to making our family function with some sense of normalcy. I am so grateful my sons always have each other.

A Sibling's Point of View

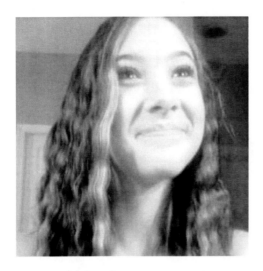

By Lydia Safford, Ben & Sam's sister

Lydia Safford is 13 years old. She lives in southern NH with her mom and her two brothers, Ben and Sam what have DMD. She also has an older step-brother named Kevin. Lydia is a talented singer and actress. When not singing and acting or at school, Lydia enjoys photography, riding her bike, playing flute, babysitting young children in her neighborhood and playing volleyball, basketball and tennis for her school. You can reach Lydia through her Facebook page, Photography by Lydia Safford.

A Sibling's Point of View

Hi, my name is Lydia Safford and this is my family story. I'm 13, and I have two brothers with Duchenne Muscular Dystrophy (DMD). Ben is 16 and Sam is 14. We live with my mom, Lori in Pelham, NH. My brothers and I go to Fellowship Christian Academy in Methuen, MA. We all go to church at Fellowship Bible Church (the same place as my school.) Sam and I are in 8th grade, and Ben is a junior in high school. Our story is a story with a lot of prayer, faith, and God's strength.

In May of 2002, our house in Windham got struck by lightning. It took 12 weeks to be fixed, so we were living in a hotel. During that time, my brothers were diagnosed with Duchenne Muscular Dystrophy. Ben was 6 and Sam was 4. My mom and dad had me tested too, to see if I was a carrier, and I am. I carry the disease, so if I have a child and it's a son, he has a 50% chance of having DMD. I feel like people don't take this seriously. It's like the disease is always going to be in my life, or has a chance to be. We finally moved back into our house and started our new life with DMD.

My mom really needed someone in a similar situation to understand what she was going through. Joan Lafferty was that person. She had two boys with DMD who were 15 and 17 at that time; she really helped my mom through this. Her younger son, Joe passed away when he was 20. And now we still hang out with Joan, her husband, Tim, and Pete who is 27. In 2004 we built an accessible home in Pelham, NH, which we still live in today. We purchased a wheelchair accessible van, and a lot of other equipment. A lot has happened since then.

My dad passed away this past January (2012). We came home from church and my mom found him; it was a totally unexpected death. It's been hardest on me, because I was the closest to him. I get so depressed when I see girls with their daddies. I just want to go back to when he was here, and I would give anything to do that. My dad was a part of me. But through this God is teaching me that I need to have a better relationship with Him. He is my real Father, and I know that He will never give up on me, no matter how much I mess up. It really comforts me to know that God is preparing a place for us with no more tears, pain, or sorrow. And I can't wait for that day to meet Jesus, my Savior. Losing my dad was really rough on my family, but God is teaching us all something through this trial. So, if you are going through something really hard right now, just know that God is always there and He has allowed this trial in your life for a reason. I know it's hard to accept that this is happening for a reason, and it took me a while to accept it too. God loves you and He's always there, no matter what. I love Him so much!

When my dad was still here, the two of us did things to get away from all the wheelchairs, and helping my brothers. On Sundays sometimes we would meet my Gramps and have breakfast with him and that was really fun. We would always stop at Dunkin Donuts and listen to the radio in the car, sing along, and make up dance moves. Yeah, he was the best daddy ever. Yes, I still call him daddy and I always will. We would do other stuff to get a break, like running errands, just daddy and me. Now my mom and I try to do things once in a while to have a break too. We go out to dinner or to the mall when a caregiver is home with the boys.

Over the summer our family wasn't together a whole lot. I went on a mission trip with my youth group to Owego, NY. That was really awesome and I had a lot of fun. The boys went to two camps for two weeks in a row. They went to the Jett Foundation camp (Camp Promise) and MDA camp. While they were at camp, my mom and I went to Cape Cod and to Ireland. It's always been a huge dream of mine (and my dad's) to go to Ireland so that was a really incredible trip. Then, close to the end of the summer, we all went to Joni and Friends Family Retreat.

Every year my mom talks to our class about DMD (Sam and I are in the same class). Last year I decided to talk to them because I thought they might be tired of hearing her every year. We watched a CureDuchenne video on Duchenne and then I spoke and sang Blessings by Laura Story. I was pretty choked up. I didn't expect that to happen. I got through the song but was in tears and right after it ended, I ran out crying. It was pretty embarrassing. I didn't expect it to be so hard to speak about what it is like to have two brothers with Duchenne, but it was. DMD affects siblings a lot too. I always think about what it would be like if they were normal--not having people stare at you, ask what happened, feel bad for you, and basically (having to) watch your siblings die. But I know I'll see them again in Heaven and that gives me hope. This world isn't our real home, and if you just believe on Jesus, He will change you forever, forgive all your sins, and give you healing--and you will have eternal life. He died for every single person in this whole world; isn't that amazing? He makes me so happy, I can't even explain it…it's indescribable. So yeah, I get depressed sometimes and angry at God for what has happened in my life, but life is way too short to spend it like that.

Ben, Sam and I went back to school on September 5th and we all enjoy it a lot. Sam plays the drums and he's really good at them. Ben sings in two choirs and he has a really awesome voice. He is also in school drama. Ben and Sam are both also in power soccer. Yes, they can play in wheelchairs, and it's really awesome. I play flute, play volleyball, tennis and basketball, I'm in school choir, and I do drama. I love singing; when I'm depressed, I put on music and sing, and it calms me down. Acting is the best thing on this earth. I love acting in plays for my town and school. Basketball is my favorite sport and I'm getting better at it. Flute is really fun to play and it sounds so beautiful. Last but not least, my mom is the best cook! She is also really good at editing, so she's editing this book.

To end, I'd like to share the lyrics from Laura Story's *Blessings* song. This song touches me in a really huge way and I can't listen to it without crying.

We pray for blessings

We pray for peace

Comfort for family, protection while we sleep

We pray for healing, for prosperity

We pray for Your mighty hand to ease our suffering

All the while, You hear each spoken need

Yet love us way too much to give us lesser things

'Cause what if your blessings come through raindrops

What if Your healing comes through tears

What if a thousand sleepless nights are what it takes to know You're near

What if trials of this life are Your mercies in disguise

We pray for wisdom

Your voice to hear

We cry in anger when we cannot feel You near

We doubt your goodness, we doubt your love

As if every promise from Your Word is not enough

All the while, You hear each desperate plea

And long that we'd have faith to believe

When friends betray us

When darkness seems to win

We know that pain reminds this heart

That this is not our home

What if my greatest disappointments

Or the aching of this life

Is the revealing of a greater thirst this world can't satisfy.

What if trials of this life

The rain, the storms, the hardest nights

Are your mercies in disguise

I would trade places with them in a heartbeat

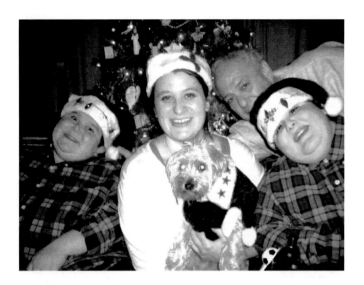

By Hope Alm

My name is Hope Alm, I am 23 years old and my brother Jackson age 16 and Hayden age 14 have Duchenne Muscular Dystrophy. I currently live in Cortland, New York, and am working as a mechanical engineer. I have never lived in the same house as Jackson and Hayden, but I have lived close most of their lives, which allowed me to be around much more often than I am able to be now.

I would trade places with them in a heartbeat

Jackson and Hayden and I all share the same father, but have different mothers. However, it was my mother and not my father who first told me that Jackson and Hayden suffered from DMD. This is one of those days that sticks out in my memory because it is the day I first learned of the devastating news. It is just like how everyone remembers where they were when JFK was killed or when the Twin Towers where struck on 911. Not a day has gone by since then that I do not think of Jackson and Hayden and how much I wish I could be around more for them. Now I live about two hours away because of my job, but of course I try to visit whenever I can.

I love to visit with Jackson and Hayden. I do not want to spend time with them just because I feel like I need to but because I honestly have a great time with them. They are funny, smart, and very entertaining kids and I enjoy every minute spent with them. Every minute I am with them is spent laughing, playing games, and making memories. These moments are the main reason I wish I could be around more. I miss them when I'm away from them.

I really do not want to get too much into how hard it is for me to see my brothers the way they are, in wheel chairs, or struggling with simple things like writing, eating or playing a game of dominoes. I do not even come close to being able to understand how hard it is not only for Jackson and Hayden, but for my Dad and their mother Diane. Although, I care very much for Jackson and Hayden and it pains me to think of how much more difficult their lives have to be because of this awful disease, it is mostly Diane and my dad who have to constantly be there for them and who are gravely affected both emotionally and physically.

Diane, who is basically my step-mom even though her and my dad have not been together for a while, is in-short, one incredible women. I am very much inspired by her strength and ability to push through the toughest of situations. I honestly do not know if I could do what she does every day if I were in her shoes. Jackson and Hayden are very fortunate to have her.

They are also very fortunate to have my father. He would do absolutely anything for his boys and he works so hard every day to make them feel special and loved, either by entering their world of fantasies or simply by playing a game with them. He is one of the hardest working men I have ever known and I realize how much time he spends just so they can feel like every other kid. He does their homework with them, he makes them laugh, and he takes them for walks. When I think of my childhood with my father, it really is not much different from that.

I know this story is supposed to bring about awareness to DMD and to explain how it affects my life as a sibling, but I really wanted to take this opportunity to state how I feel about Jackson and Hayden's mother, Diane, and my father, Robert and how amazingly they take care of those boys, each in their individual ways. Both Diane and my dad wrote a story of their own in *"Saving Our Sons and Daughters II"*, which is how I became aware of the opportunity to tell my story.

I guess to simply state how DMD has specifically affected my life; I would say that although my brothers have it, they are not defined by it. When I think of them, I think of how much fun I have just playing a game of dominoes with them and I appreciate the fact that they are two amazing kids. I would trade places with them in a heartbeat if I could or if I could magically take the disease from them I would, but I would not trade them for any other brothers in the entire world, with or without DMD.

For Hope

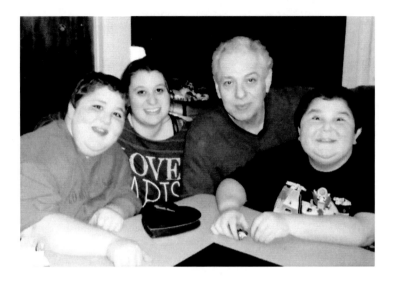

By: Bob Alm

My name is Bob, spelled the same frontwards and backwards, a palindrome, much like "A man a plan a canal Panama." I am currently engaged to a wonderful woman named Marilyn, who I have been with for nearly Fourteen years. I have three children, a Twenty-Three year old daughter, Hope, born on April Third; her mother's name is Karen. I also have two boys, Jackson, who is Seventeen as of December Fourth, and Hayden who is fifteen as of June Ninth. Both of my sons have Duchene's Muscular Dystrophy. They were diagnosed at around age two or three. All three of my children are great kids. At age Fifty-Four, I am pleased to have three such gifted offspring. Hope graduated from R.I.T. with an Engineering degree, last year and she currently works for Intertek Corp. in Cortland. Jackson is in Eleventh grade, while Hayden is in Ninth. Both are still in main stream high school, taking college preparation courses. I have been a business man for over thirty years. I was a regional supervisor of Burger King Restaurants, owned my own restaurant/tavern, was in the vending business, and was a registered nurse for five years. Currently, I am self-employed owning rental properties and doing remodeling of homes. I work when I want to now, not when I have to. I am not wealthy; I just have other priorities to think about.

For Hope

There is a song that used to be sung every year during the Labor Day Telethon; sometimes by Jerry Lewis, sometimes by Jack Johnson, called "If I Could." Although I worked the Telethon growing up, I never really paid much attention to it; until my sons were diagnosed with Muscular Dystrophy. After that, it quickly became my favorite song, although I cried my eyes out, the first time that I paid attention to the words. My favorite version of the song was recorded by Ray Charles; (it is readily available on I-tunes, you should give it a listen if you get the chance.) The lyrics say everything that a parent or sibling of a child with a debilitating disease feels, as a matter of fact, now that I think of it, it invokes the feelings that any parent of any child feels, if they are truly a parent. That being said, I have it on my I-pod and I have made numerous discs with that particular version of the song on the playlists. I never listen to them. It hurts too much. Much like cracked crab legs, my favorite food, (and the one thing that I am allergic to in life,) it remains my favorite, although I never eat it; and I never listen to the song. You see, it reminds me not only of my sons and the adversity that they face, every day, but more so of the adversities that I face, and worse still; it reminds me most of my daughter, Hope.

Now adversity is a part of everyone's life, rich or poor, educated or ignorant, but let's face it, some people have it worse than others. They say what doesn't kill you makes you stronger. I hate that phrase; partly because it is so cliché, but mostly because most of the time, I would much rather have it kill me than to have to deal with it. Now, don't get me wrong, I do not want to die, this isn't some latent death wish or the ravings of a person with clinical depression or something, but I have to ask myself sometimes; what kind of a plan is it that God has for my family, that so much adversity can be poured out on to those so young and undeserving of it. As for myself, I have not lived the life that I expected and the adversity that I face, (with the exception of my three children,) has for the most part, been brought upon myself by me, and I deserve some of it.

I have said before that I am not proud of my past. From the time I hit the age of Twenty, I chose to ignore what was important in life. It took many years and a number of divorces to teach me again, that family was the most important thing in life. Now that I have learned that lesson, it seems that its inherent benefits are to be ripped from me, well before their time. When I go to Church, I feel like everyone in the room is asking God, "Whens it gonna rain?" I feel like screaming out, "When's it gonna stop?" At any rate, when I hear the song, all that I can think about is my children. First I think of my boys and then my thoughts immediately turn to my daughter and the adversities that she has already faced in life and of those yet to come.

Let me tell you about Hope. She is a young woman now, out on her own for the first time, living in another town, working her first real full-time job as an engineer. She is Twenty-Three now, and has already completed college and pursued a career. Hope is the most intelligent, funny, thoughtful, and beautiful girl that I have ever known; and she is my daughter! I would like to tell you that she got it all from me, but I would be lying. Her mother is just as smart, just as beautiful, and just as funny as Hope. I am none of the above.

Hope shares other traits with her mom though that are wonderful, but sometimes can be a burden. You see, she is also extremely sensitive, loves deeply, and she cares very much about everything that is important. It shames me sometimes that she shares some of my traits as well. I am a cynic, a pragmatist, and I am very intolerant of the shortcomings of others. I try to see the world as it is and it saddens me to see what I do. Unfortunately, this has rubbed off on Hope. You would think that I would be proud that I have prepared her for what life holds in store for her, but I am afraid that all that I have done is to take away her innocence and replace it with my jaded view of the world. Hope enters the world as a free spirit without the naivety that would make all of her experiences wonderful and new. Although this is comforting to me, (the lack of naivety I mean,) I fear that I have robbed her of some experiences that will now cause her to worry instead of embracing the situation and moving forward without regrets. If this is the case, then I say here, for the record, Honey, I am sorry, truly. The truth is that I worry for her more than my boys. I guess that is because at the very least, they can see what's coming. As for my daughter, I have no clue.

Hope has known about Jackson and Hayden's disease since they were diagnosed. She understands only too well what it means for their future. Although she has a different mother, Hope has been as good a sister to my sons, as any sibling could be. While she was growing up, we spent as much time together as possible, (the four of us, I mean.) While she was in school, she made it a point to come over on Tuesdays and Thursdays when I had the boys, in order to spend time and play games with them. They interact much as any other siblings do, playing and fighting together, playfully picking on each other's faults, sharing private jokes, and cutting down their father. I have found these to be some of the most rewarding days of my life. Even now, while she lives three hours away, Hope makes the time to come over and spend time with her brothers, every time she comes home. I know that like myself, she enjoys every minute that she spends with her siblings, and that like me, she worries about their future.

I am worried about what the future will bring though, as the disease progresses in my boys. Jackson is Seventeen now and Hayden fifteen. It will not be long, (unless, God willing, a cure is found,) that the seriousness of their condition will manifest itself. I don't even know how I am going to handle these times yet, even though I have worked with DMD patients in the hospital before as a nurse, and I know what to expect. Hope has faced so much already for someone so young; the death of an Uncle who was only as old as her parents, the loss of Conner, my Grandson, who she absolutely adored, and countless other adversities, (not least of which are the problems that her father has had.) I do not wish any more on her. On that note, I have a message for her and my boys; it's the lyrics to the Ray Charles song, "If I Could."

Hope,

If I could- I'd protect you from the sadness in your eyes. Give you courage in a world of compromise.

Yes I would…

If I could- I would teach you all the things I never learned. And I'd help you cross the bridges that I've burned.

Yes I would…

If I could- I would try to shield your innocence from time. But the part of life I gave you isn't mine. I watched you grow- so that I could let you go…

If I could- I would help you make it through the hungry years. But I know that I could never dry your tears.

But I would- If I could…

Yes, if I live- in a time and place where you don't want to be, you don't have to walk along this road with me. My yesterday- won't have to be your way…

If I knew- I would try to change the world I brought you to. And there isn't very much that I could do.

But I would- If I could…

Oh, baby, daddy want's to protect you- and help my baby through the hungry years. "Cause your part of me. And if you ever, ever need a shoulder to cry on, or just someone to talk to, I'll be there, I'll be there. I didn't change the world.

But I would- If I could…

"Oh darlin'. I love you baby."

Mama Bear & Sissy

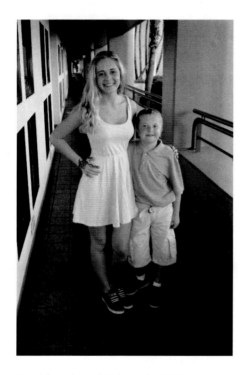

By Sherri and Victoria Ritter

Nicholas Ritter Son and Brother is 9 years old and was diagnosed with Duchenne in March of 2011 Being a voice for your child or brother is a strong way to advocate for the disease that could so crucially change your lives forever. Visit You Tube Nicholas Ritter's Seal of Courage: Music by Orianthi…

A Parent's Point of View

When your child gets diagnosed with a fatal disease that has no cure, you immediately go into "Mama Bear" mode. This means that you will do whatever it takes to protect him. Some of us might even be known as a "smothering Mama Bear", like me for instance. If I can offer any words of advice to any parent who might be living through the nightmare of a Duchenne diagnosis, it would be: "let him be a child for as long as he can, act like there is no disease". Basically, treat him as normally as possible, allowing him to live without any inhibitions. I may repeat this statement throughout the story, but that is because I still have to keep reminding myself of it on a daily basis.

The moment you hear those words "It's Duchenne", it's a whole new ball game. You're asking if it could be Becker or Limb Girdle. You're thinking "if it is Muscular Dystrophy, please God let it be the lesser of the evils." Not that there really is a *better* one. When I received the news about Nicholas, I immediately went into "save my son mode" and my 14-year-old daughter got put on the sidelines. She was good, right? She didn't have a terminal disease. It was about a year later when I realized that Nicholas was essentially getting away with everything short of murder and my daughter Tori was being punished for everything she did wrong and that I was not encouraging her for all the positive things she did. The realization came after their father and I were divorced. She finally said "you don't care about me, it's all about Nick, and by the way Mom, you're creating a monster". It was then that I realized that although Nicholas has a disease, he is still responsible for all his actions. Just because he was considered terminally ill, I should not have been treating him like an abnormal child.

As a mother it was tough to treat him normally because I always wanted to protect him from harm and Duchenne is certainly a major threat. I wanted to spend every minute, no, every second with him, but I realized that I would suffocate him. He could not flourish or experience life if I did that. This quote was posted on my Facebook Page and it made me think: "Enjoy today and always hold hope for tomorrow because some day tomorrow will be today." I now feel empowered to continue fighting this disease. My DMD family has really inspired me to never give up hope no matter what the situation. This whole experience has made me stronger.

My daughter Victoria has always been a bright, funny, outgoing, *life of the party* kind of child. She is not shy by any means. Once I fought my way out of my bubble, I realized how withdrawn and unhappy she had become. Sure, she had her moments, but they were few and far between.

What I didn't realize was that she was feeling the same as I rejected, withdrawn, and fearful. The fear of the unknown, what was going to happen to Nick, how much time do we have with him? Is it OK to fight with my brother? Every time she did, I would get upset and say enjoy the time you have, but now I know without that without sibling rivalry they had an unhealthy relationship. So go ahead and fight, I'm going into the other room. What I did notice is that in her idle time,. Victoria (Sissy) was there for her brother. She had patience when he had outbursts; she helped calm him down during difficult times. She is his sissy and always will be. My wish is that she would have the same passion as I do to be an advocate and to help with fundraisers and shout out to everyone that this is Duchenne, this is my brother and let's fight this disease together. I now know not to push her into becoming the person I want to be, she is only a teenager! I am now surrounded by a strong support group of friends and family. I especially want to thank my close friend Scott for always being in the battle with me from the beginning. I will fight this disease no matter what and do what it takes to protect both of my children and stop DMD from being passed down from one generation to another.

Tori's Story

"Stronger"

Hi, I'm Tori Ritter. I'm fifteen years old and my brother, Nick, was diagnosed with DMD in March of 2011when he was 7 years old. Before Duchenne, I was a happy exuberant, loud, and athletic young teenage girl. After Duchenne my life was changed forever.

I remember the day that we found out about Nick's diagnosis. It was the day of my hockey team's party. My dad had received a phone call saying Nick had Muscular Dystrophy and from then on, it was complete chaos. About two months later, we found out it was Duchenne and a month after that my parents filed for what turned into a divorce.

Like I said, my life did a complete 180. Everything happened back to back, it was just like a continuing smack to the face. Once you got back up again, you were pushed right back to the ground. At least that's what it felt like to me. I was on the Internet all day and slept all night. My bedroom was my escape from reality and my dreams were the only place I could be free. I didn't know it at the time, but I was becoming clinically depressed. I was withdrawing from the world around me. I didn't want to play hockey anymore, I hid from my family for numerous hours, I would lie when my friends asked to hangout and say that my mom wouldn't let me.

At this point in my home life, Nick had yet to visit Cincinnati Children's Hospital and start his steroid treatment and my dad had moved out of my house. It was a total adjustment for me, and I don't accept change very well. I didn't want to stress my parents out anymore by telling them that I was struggling with an eating disorder, but the teachers told them anyway.

By this time Nick had started his new medications and I was getting ready to start high school. My high school had all accelerated classes which would ultimately cut about two years off of college. That meant 10 months of school, many sleepless nights, and so much homework that you didn't even know where to start. As you can tell, I was already in enough distress from everything else. School was the cherry to top it all off. I had mental breakdowns at least twice a week from the stress, from the anxiety, from the perfectionist that lived inside me. Eventually I just gave up and I didn't do my homework.

I was familiar with the new medication Nick was on because when I was young and had asthma I was on steroids too. I knew about the swollen face and eating all the time. What I didn't remember was the "Roid Rage" as they call it. Nicholas turned into a screaming, ranting and raving maniac. What I thought was some down home sibling rivalry was actually the steroids in full force. He was hitting me and always screaming and yelling. Most people thought it was Nicholas being bad but my mom and I knew it wasn't. My dad would just refuse to deal with it and Nick was getting away with everything with my mom just because she wanted to keep him quiet. I would hear her cry at night wanting to do the right thing, but it was going to be a slow change.

Every morning that I spend with my brother the anxiety sets in, and I ask myself, "will he be ok today"? "Is he going to fall"?

"What can I do to make him better?" "It is a never-ending battle." I want this all to go away; this cure cannot come quick enough. I love my brother. My other fear is that one day when I get older I will have kids of my own. Will they have this disease? What can I do to prevent it? No child of my age or of my brother's should ever have to ask themselves that question. That is why I am going to do what I can and work with my mom to be an advocate and join this network that is so fighting very hard to find a cure for this disease.

Our home life has stabilized and we have come to terms with the fact that DMD in in our lives to stay. We are in a positive stride. Nicholas has not deteriorated too much since his diagnosis, so it's difficult to visualize the future. For now its one day at a time with my brother and the D word (Duchenne). My mom tries to do all that she can and I know some days are really tough for her with Nicholas's mood swings. I usually make her take a time out and I try to be patient with Nicholas because I can only imagine how frustrated he gets.

Duchenne has changed my life; there is no doubt about it. There is one thing I will *not* let it change though: my future. I am a fighter, so is my brother, my mom, and my dad. We are all battling our inner fears. I plan to do something with my life and not simply sit and mope around, complaining about it all the time. I **will** make a difference, I **will** find a cure, and I **will not** let this disease bring me down that low again. No, **I am *so* much stronger than that**.

An Amazing Love

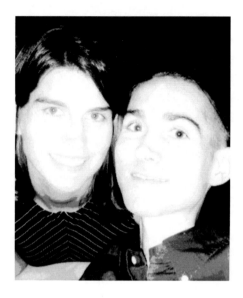

By Jeannine (Rowe) Sawvel

Jeannine (Rowe) Sawvel grew up in Michigan. She pursued a Bachelor's Degree from Grand Valley State University and completed her Masters in Early Childhood Education. She was a Special Education teacher for eight years before choosing to stay home with her daughters. She has a huge passion for the great outdoors and adventure. Her family remains her number one priority in life. Jeannine resides in Minnesota with her husband, Jay, and their two daughters, Mackenzie and Miranda.

An Amazing Love

My brother Steven was my best friend. Words cannot even begin to explain the love and bond we shared! He was one of the most remarkable people I have ever known; I am not sure I have ever loved anyone else so deeply. Nor, I have never before or since spent seventeen years loving someone I knew was dying. It is different…it just is different.

Steven was diagnosed with Duchenne Muscular Dystrophy (DMD) at age four. I was eight years old at the time. I remember the moment my mom told me. I don't recall her exact words, but I remember a box of Kleenex and sobbing. At that moment I became fully aware that my little brother was eventually going to be wheelchair bound and then one day die. There was nothing I could do to change that; it was inevitable. After that day we never really talked again about Steven dying. My mom stood firm making his life as "normal" as possible, and he would be given as many opportunities as we could possibly give him. We were going to hope and pray for a miracle in the meantime.

As Steven grew up his body progressively failed him, but he never let that stop him from having fun. Our lives were filled with swimming, wheelchair races, friends and adventure! Steven loved being with family, had a huge passion for cars, especially old ones, and was a gifted artist. He was an adorable little boy who grew into an inspiring teenager and a remarkable young man. His determination and ability to adapt took him great places. His amazing artwork won numerous awards, and his story was told over and over again in the newspaper. When DMD crept in and stole his ability to paint, Steven didn't stop. Instead, he created his own business. He developed his own website where he sold prints of his paintings and other artists' work as well. High School graduation came and went, and I bawled like a baby, being ever so proud to be his sister. Then college and eventually the day I had dreaded my entire life…his death. Steven died on March 28, 2000, at the age of 21, with my mom and me by his side.

Growing up on the sidelines of DMD made me different. People didn't look at me differently, but my thoughts and life concerns were completely different than other children around me. My biggest worry as a teenager was not what I looked like, but would I be with Steven when he died. How would I assure that I was? That thought was a consuming, constant fear. Right up until the moment he died that was my biggest concern in life. My number one priority was making sure he did not die alone. It didn't stop me from going off to college and having fun, but it was always present in my mind. That was a tremendous weight to carry as a child and even into adulthood; it was a burden I quickly realized I could not control.

Living with someone who is terminally ill can trigger cyclical grief. This is where you grieve over and over again continuously until that day you dreaded your whole life comes, and your loved one dies. Then you enter a different journey of grief. Essentially even though my brother did not die until I was 25, I grieved his loss from the early age of eight. Seventeen years of watching, waiting and wondering how it was all going to end. That is what siblings are forced to face. The totality of this experience has made me a deeply compassionate person, one who feels another's pain to the depth of my core, one who believes there is nothing, nothing, more important than family.

Living a childhood intertwined with grief made my outlook on life more complicated than my peers. I am a very logical, realistic thinker. It is hard to look at the "glass as half full" when you are dealt a hand of such enormous emotional challenges. Positive and hopeful on the surface for my brother, but at age thirteen I could not find anything positive about watching my nine year old brother lose his ability to walk. To this day it is still very difficult to adopt the "glass half full" attitude. I am just way too realistic and that is hard sometimes.

I never wanted anyone to experience my emotional pain but so badly wanted one person to understand what I was going through. The good times were great, at which times I felt no different than any other member of a "normal" family. However, the times of struggle and exhaustion watching my mom (who was an amazing mom and caregiver), or watching Steven, quickly reminded me that our life was anything but "normal." I felt alone. I craved normalcy.

All parents need to be aware that yes, siblings feel guilt, and for some it is overpowering. Siblings are often overlooked - it is understandable in the big picture as the disease takes its toll. But it is true. We siblings, especially male siblings I think, feel guilt because we ourselves do not have the disease. For some it is more overpowering than others and needs to be addressed. This is not something I struggled with but my older brother, David, was heavily burdened with this guilt.

The possibility of being a carrier was another challenge I faced. Personally, this was another weight on my young shoulders well before I should have been preoccupied with thoughts of having children. I remember when I decided to undergo genetic testing. The doctor looked at me and said, "Why are you even worried about this? You are not married or looking to have children right now." I was appalled at his ignorance. That is exactly why it was on my mind. I had to know before I met the man who would steal my heart. I had to know because for me, if I was a carrier, I would have chosen to adopt rather than have biological children. To make a long story short, I was not a carrier. I thank God for that blessing.

Living with a brother who had DMD directly impacted my career choice. I have a huge heart, the determination to make a difference and a huge sense of hope. I pursued a degree in Psychology/Special Education and went on to become a teacher. My number one choice for a classroom was teaching children who had severe multiple impairments. My students were amazing, and it didn't take me long to become their advocate! I believed in them and I could relate to their parents, most of whom were in a grieving process of their own. It was easier for me to relate to these parents than to my own peers. Nobody I knew at twenty-three understood grief; I still run into that problem with my peers today. Making a difference in someone else's world was so rewarding! I felt like I was finally able to give back for all of those wonderful people who gave so much to my brother.

The final days of Steven's life could fill the pages of a book all on their own. What an amazing, heart-wrenching, exhausting and beautiful experience. Nothing teaches you more about life than death. Nothing secured my faith more than being with him when he died. I was so relieved for him that he was finally free of DMD but yet so immensely heartbroken for myself. Nothing could have prepared me for how much I was going to miss him. It broke my heart to the depths of my inner being. I cried for what felt like weeks and months. I felt alone, trying to hide my enormous pain from my mom, who was in the middle of her own grief. When you lose a sibling you honestly do lose a piece of yourself. You grieve the loss of your brother or sister and you grieve the loss of yourself, for you will never be the same person after that moment. I was not quite aware that I would suddenly be confused about where I fell in the birth order. Nor had I ever thought about how I would answer the question, "Do you have siblings?" "Yes, yes I do. I have two brothers" and then the look on people's faces and their sudden lack for words when you tell them one is deceased. Awkward only begins to describe the sudden turn in conversation. But in time, as I have healed, answering those questions became easier. I became more confident in my answer and proud of how far I had come in my own healing.

Learning to live without Steven was difficult. I wanted him back so badly. The first year was rough with all the firsts: the first birthday, the first Christmas the first everything without him. But as time passes your tears become fewer and the time between tears becomes greater. The hole in your heart is never repaired, but the pain becomes less severe. Life distracts you, and you find a new normal. I got married several years after Steven died and gave birth to two beautiful girls. Steven is still a huge part of their lives even though they have never met him. The older one has his artistic talent and the younger one his big brown eyes! We continue to celebrate Steven's birthday every year because a birthday is a celebration of a life and his life most definitely should be celebrated!

Steven and his life were my biggest blessings! DMD affected us both in different ways, but neither one of us ever let the horrific disease define us. Steven never let the disease win. Every time it stole from him he fought back harder. Even when his heart was functioning at only 5 %, he got up every single day and went to class. He never used the disease as an excuse. His attitude toward life, his determination to succeed and his passion for art were inspiring to everyone around him. Nothing was more important to Steven than his family and friends. He was extremely loyal, the best listener and simply the best friend anyone could hope for. He was a true inspiration of how one should live his or her life. He loved people to the depth of his soul and taught the rest of us to do the same. He smiled every single day, no matter what. He was a gift, a precious gift to all those who were lucky enough to have known him. There is no question I am a better person because of him. I feel so incredibly blessed to have been part of his life. What a gift to have been able to experience his entire journey with him. I am completely honored to be his sister.

I firmly believe there is a greater purpose for all that I have endured. There is a reason why I was chosen to be Steven's sister. There is a greater purpose for all the pain and heartbreak. All these years later I am still discovering what that purpose is, but writing this story is definitely part of it. No one sitting on the sidelines of DMD should ever feel alone. We are all in this together. We need to join hands and fight back. Our brothers and sisters, you and me, we are all the prime examples of strength and the ability to overcome. We need to reach out and support one another in this journey. DMD stole from us all, but it also made us the compassionate, strong, determined survivors that we are. It gave us all the very tools we need to band together, advocate, fight back and eventually destroy this horrific disease forever.

In memory of all those who have gone before us, in honor of those who are currently in the fight and to all of us on the sidelines-may we never let this disease define us, may we never give up hope, and may we never lose sight of our ability to love to the depths of our souls.

My brother John

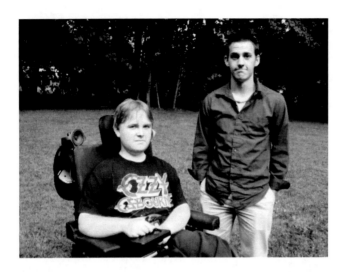

By Michael Norton

My name is Michael Norton and I live in Standish, Maine. I am 24 years of age, living with Duchenne Muscular Dystrophy. I haven't let this disease slow me down. Some of the things that I am into are graphic design, art, editing videos, skateboarding, football, hockey, zombies, women, beer and heavy metal music. I'm taking courses at a local community college in the field of Communications and New Media. In my spare time I often draw with Adobe Illustrator, edit YouTube videos and blast death metal tunes. I like my music loud, fast, brutal and when the vocals are screaming. I am also a trend setter and somewhat of a fashion designer. My hopes with my company, Disabledcrip Industries, is to get my name out there and show people that just because you're in a wheelchair doesn't mean you have to follow the rules. I am a hell raising rebel at heart. Since I have a creative mind, I find no down time. My brain consistently works overtime on new and crazy ideas. I can never stop creating. I am in the process of opening a little store on my website with my T-shirt designs and other art endeavors. I am known as the Heavy Metal Cripple within the YouTube community. I often make videos covering topics such as the latest heavy metal releases or myself doing ridiculous outlandish things like drinking and swearing. Bands often get in touch with me and send me their CDs to review. It's a pretty good gig as life is full of surprises.

My brother John

My brother John has always helped me with many obstacles I have faced. Without him, I wouldn't know what to do. He is a big part of who I am. We are close in age. Our lives haven't been anything out of the ordinary. We would get into trouble like most brothers. Growing up, we had a lot of the same friends. When we were younger, he felt obligated to look out for me at school. Sometimes there would be conflicts with other kids because he thought they were trying to hurt us. My brother and I both went through a lot of anger. I went through a lot of anger because of what was happening to my body. My brother was angry because he had a hard time watching me get weaker. I remember my mom brought us to counselors.

Throughout the years our house was filled with friends. My mom used to host movie night and all our friends would sleep overnight. When we were in high school, we would go skateboarding and raise heck and make videos together. He would film a lot of the scenes and some of our friends also filmed. I would edit the videos. He always tried to include me. Sometimes it was difficult because they would all take off and get into cars and I couldn't go with them. When my brother got his license, he drove me in our van and we would travel with our road crew going to skate parks around the state. I felt like a normal person who was able to do a lot of things with friends. Having a brother who was able bodied opened a lot of doors for me. He helped to make me comfortable in my own skin. We both had girlfriends at the same time. I felt normal- like I didn't have a terminal disease.

One time my parents went away for the weekend to Massachusetts. They told us we could have three or four close friends over and to behave. My brother was in charge of my care. No parents should give any teenager that freedom. We decided to do some of that stuff, except we threw the good behavior part out the window. Our friends came over to stay overnight. We were responsible and did not drive anywhere. I bought a thirty pack of beer. We thought we got away with it, until my mom later went down cellar and found a bag under the stairs with a brand of beer she did not recognize. Several of the beer cans had straws still in them. This was just one of our funny antics. There are a lot more that we just can't talk about.

My brother is a good brother. He brought me to a few metal concerts even though he is not a huge fan of that genre of music. Dying Fetus is a death metal band. My brother drove me to that concert in Manchester, NH. We went into the mosh pit and some kid slid into my wheelchair and sliced his eyebrow. One time I went to another concert which was Job for a Cowboy. We took a friend and we ended up at the hospital. We were driving home, when I couldn't breathe from CO_2 build-up in my lungs. I went in and out of consciousness and our friend alerted my brother who was driving. My brother drove like a madman to the hospital running through red lights. I somehow was able to drive into the hospital. When I was there, they gave me oxygen and an IV.

My brother was so concerned about me that he didn't realize his face was swollen from a kick to the face when he was near the mosh pit. He fractured some bones in his face. Luckily we were able to come home late that evening. My brother saved my life that night.

Another time we drove to Rye, NH, to an indoor skate park. I was getting over a cold and we did not bring the cough assist machine with us. My CO_2 levels were building up again and I struggled to breathe. My brother called an ambulance. When the ambulance arrived, I lost consciousness. My brother insisted on joining me in the ambulance. He tried to tell the doctors that I needed a cough assist machine treatment, but they wouldn't listen. They ended up intubating me and catheterizing me. They asked my brother to get out of the room when I was intubated. My brother refused to leave. Nobody was listening to us. They transferred me by ambulance to Maine Medical Center. Afterwards, my brother had to take a cab to get back to the van to drive back to Maine. He didn't have enough money but after talking with the cab driver about the experience, the driver revealed that he also had a form of muscular dystrophy. He understood the circumstances and excused my brother's lack of funds. Again, my brother saved my life. I felt bad that he wasn't able to skateboard that day. We were both very angry about the experience, and did not speak about it or see each other until a day had passed.

We are still very close, as my brother has been my caregiver for a few years. Sometimes, I feel like a burden and I feel like I am holding him back from life. Brothers are important and we learn from each other. We may get frustrated but in the end we are brothers and we will always figure it out and have a laugh or two about it in the end. We stick together.

A Poem for my brother,

By Pete Lafferty

Pete is a 26-year old young man with Duchenne. He lives with his family in Nashua, NH, and enjoys writing poetry, speaking, and serving as emcee at Joni and Friends New England Family Retreats.

Joey Lafferty

9/22/1987 - 11/18/2007

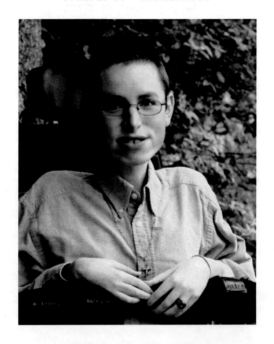

A POEM FOR MY BROTHER

You were quite a bro

And you let it show

You were always super courageous

With a smile that was contagious

All of you Joe loved

And he flew like a dove

He now soars like an eagle

Not like an ordinary sea gull

You we will miss

And we'll blow you a kiss

You were so brave

And not death's slave

You were quite a joy

Ever since you were a little boy

From a special friend you loved a hug

With your Red Sox blanket you were snug

You loved dogs and cats

And looked cool in hats

You liked the Pats

And rooted for those guys with the Red Sox caps

Now when I see a rainbow

I'll think of God's promise to you

You now have eternal life

And no more strife

You are the champ

And we loved going to Joni Camp

You're now in heaven

And it's you we're craving

You were so good

And you sure enjoyed food

You were never in a bad mood

You loved meeting babies

Your new life is sweeter than candies

You lived life with such grace

And now you've won the race

Oh how we miss you so

You were quite a bro

By: Pete Lafferty

Ashley...

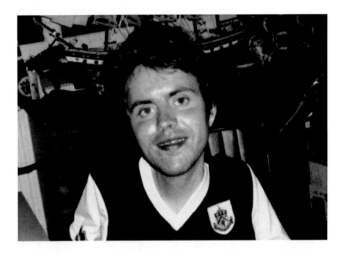

By Maggy Simpson

I am 24 years old. My brother Ashley Adam Kirkham had Duchenne Muscular Dystrophy and was sadly taken away from us on 18th February 2010 aged 27 Years. Ashley started to write a book about the condition and how it affected him - I would like to finish the book in memory of him. Tilted; *'Through thick and thin, A life with Duchenne.'* As I cannot say it from his point of view it will be a sibling's point of view which is also where the poems come in. This condition has a great impact on everyone, as it did with all our family. The pain and hurt we still feel so raw even after nearly a year. My poems are a way to express the way the condition affects those who have it and their families, but also try to get the reader understanding that although these boys/men have this condition they are still normal people with normal everyday feelings.

I sit here now and I wonder,

Wonder if things will improve,

Wonder if a cure will be found,

Before more people have to lose.

The pain these people go through,

I cannot comprehend.

I wish that there was something I could do,

Something more then lend a hand.

People need to realize, and people need to learn too.

I saw it through my brothers eyes, and this I share with you.

A boy trapped inside a shell, a boy that had dreams,

A boy who never thought of himself, a boy that was never mean.

He was an angel sent down to us,

Sent so we could be aware,

Aware that through all this pain, we still had love to share.

Sent to help us realize, and sent to give us hope, too,

That someday in the future, their suffering will be through.

~Maggy Simpson

In memory of Ashley Adam Kirkham who had Duchenne Muscular Dystrophy.

My Brother Patrick

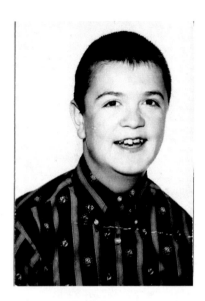

By Geri Karlin

Geri Karlin is a Registered Nurse with 20 years of experience. She is the mother of four: Lauren, Brittany, Cassidy and Ryan. She has been married to her husband Marty for 19 years. Her brother Patrick was 17 when he died as a result of Duchenne Muscular Dystrophy. Her son Ryan was diagnosed with Duchenne on April 15, 2008.He is now 10 years old. She started a charity with her husband in 2009 called Rally for Ryan. They have raised over $500,000 for Duchenne Research and Awareness. Her hope is to prevent this disease from taking another family member far too soon.

My Brother Patrick

I was walking with my childhood friend across the street from my childhood house and she asked me when my brother Patrick was coming home from the hospital? I replied that he should be home soon, as he was getting better. Little did I know my brother would not be coming home. He had Duchenne Muscular Dystrophy. He died at age 17.

I was 6 years old on the day he died, November 8, 1970. I turned 7 six days later. I was young but I remember it as though it were yesterday. Patrick was my oldest brother, then came my brother, - who was 15, my sister, who was 12, and me, who was the middle girl, age 7, and my youngest sister, who was 18 months old. She never really knew my brother because she was a baby when he died.

I remember my mother and father getting everything ready for the funeral. A month earlier my mother had put a beautiful brown plaid fur coat and hat on lay-away at the clothing store. It was a bittersweet moment getting a beautiful new coat for such a sad occasion. I hate plaid to this day. The funeral was at St. Ferdinand's Church in Chicago. My brother was so young; the whole parish attended his services. I was a Brownie in the Girl Scouts, and I remember sitting in the first pew as everyone I knew passed us by with such sad looks and sad eyes, People were crying, but trying not to. I know it sounds strange but somehow I felt embarrassed and somewhat ashamed. I only thought I would be known in school as the little girl whose brother died.

My brother Patrick was in a wheelchair since third grade. What can I say about Duchenne Muscular Dystrophy? It's a robber of all muscle function. First your core muscles begin to weaken, then your chest protrudes to accommodate for balance. Then you begin to fall frequently but you can't get up right away. Boys with DMD struggle with all their might to stand up. But they persevere. The stairs become roadblocks which they are unable to climb due to their lack of strength and balance. It makes it nearly impossible for them to get around. They surrender a little at a time until they are in a wheelchair full time. I have actually heard from some boys who said the wheelchair helped them keep up with their friends because it made them mobile again. Can you imagine a wheelchair making you mobile again?

My brother attended a special school in Chicago named Spaulding. It was a school for children with special needs. My dad had to build a ramp in the yard to get my brother in and out of the house. My mom would take Patrick down the ramp every day to get him to the school bus. My brother Thomas would hurry home from school to help my mom care for Patrick. When he got older my dad was at work when the bus came.

Because my brother attended Spaulding he met several boys with the same illness.

My brother's friends were always upbeat, although they were also affected with Duchenne. I remember one of the moms was always crying, another mom was very angry all the time, another mom prayed a lot, but my mom always tried to be upbeat. All the boys would hang out and have fun. When I think about it now it was like a combination support/play group, which was revolutionary at the time in the 60's. They all passed away within a couple of years of one another.

It was hard on my mom and dad. The daily care was intense; one can only imagine. Patrick needed help with all activities of daily living--showering, toileting, dressing, eating, drinking and school work. They had to put special shoes on Patrick with braces in them. Just getting a drink of water required help. But I mostly remember my brother Patrick sitting in his wheelchair with a card table in front of him watching the White Sox and the Packers.

I remember being in the limo on the way to the cemetery feeling like I was going to get sick. My brother Tom gave me a piece of gum which seemed to help. After the cemetery everyone came back to our house. My mom and dad's bed had so many coats on it they reached the ceiling. I remember being in the corner of the room crying so no one would see me. It was the only place in our house not filled with people. And then it was over.

Going back to school the next day was awful but when I look back on it now, my mom and dad probably needed time to figure out what to do next. When your first born baby goes to heaven and you are left behind you push forward for everyone.

After all this, I was just a six-year-old girl waiting for my seventh birthday in four days on November 14. I don't remember my actual birthday party that year. I remember the sadness around me and turning seven just came and went; I thought 8 will be better. That spring I also made my communion; my parents tried to make it happy but that too was really hard on my mom and dad. My brother was gone forever. Our family had a new dynamic. -Survival.

As we were growing up we really didn't talk about Patrick too much because it was still very sad. Although my parents were relieved that he was no longer suffering and in pain, they missed him terribly.

Every year we watched the Jerry Lewis Muscular Dystrophy Telethon on Labor Day weekend and hoped for a cure so no one would have to suffer what our family and many others did. My dad would go in the basement and call the telethon and tell him our story and he would cry. I think he thought if we didn't see him we wouldn't know he was crying.

Over the years as time started to heal my mom and dad, they would share stories with us:

One story they told was when my brother attended MDA Camp around age 9. My mom tells of her and my dad picking Pat up at the bus from camp. A fireman volunteer carried Pat off the bus and handed him to my parents and said he no longer walks. My mom asked Pat what was wrong and he said that he couldn't keep up with the other kids so they put him in a wheelchair. And that was that, my brother no longer could walk. Keep in mind we didn't even own a wheelchair. My parent's landlord gave my dad a stroller he rigged up to put him in until they could get to the MDA clinic. There still was no treatment and no cure, not much was really known yet about this terminal debilitating disease.

When my mom was expecting me they visited the MDA clinic. The nurse behind the desk looked over her glasses at my mom and said "you're pregnant... I hope that baby will be OK". The disappointed look from the nurse said it all. They wanted the pregnancy terminated which was not an option for my mom. She had a strong faith and knew it would turn out fine. After I was born they checked me at the clinic and told my mom I was just fine, no worries. The only problem was they were wrong as I would find out many years later.

I am the mother of twin girls named Lauren and Brittany; Cassidy came three years later. I then suffered a stillborn baby boy named Jordan Rafferty who had anencephaly and never made it. My heart and world was broken, my husband and I had to recover this unimaginable loss. And we somehow did.

Then I got pregnant with my son Ryan. The amount of joy we had could hardly be contained. We hoped and prayed for a healthy happy baby. I never did find out the sex of any of my babies because I think it's one of the few surprises left in life.

On June 20, 2002, Ryan made his appearance into the world. It was one of the happiest day of my life once again, because he was a happy healthy baby. Ryan was a normal baby boy who reached all of his milestones on time. He was just a very gentle, kind child. Never having a boy before, we didn't realize until he was about 5 that he seemed a little weak. Ryan had large calves but could walk just fine. I took him to the doctor to get a blood test but deep down in my gut I knew something was terribly wrong. But having been told I was not a carrier, I didn't think the unthinkable could be possible.

On April 15, 2008, the most unimaginable test result came back. Ryan's CPK was 25,000; normal is 250. My baby had Duchenne Muscular Dystrophy.

I will never forget thinking of that nurse who told my mother I was just fine, I was not a carrier, not to worry. They told her my older sister was a carrier and it's a 50/50 chance that she might have a Duchenne baby. She never got rechecked and she played Russian roulette, but her son was fine. I was lucky or so I thought. My sisters both had boys that were unaffected and I never thought this could happen to my son. I assumed the previous information given to me was true and correct. Then DNA testing became available but it was too late, my only son Ryan was diagnosed with Duchenne Muscular Dystrophy at age 5. So my whole life has been dealing with the effects of Duchenne and I now have to live with Duchenne again until I leave this world.

After all those years of watching my mom and dad care for my brother, I decided long ago that I wanted to become a nurse. Watching their love and commitment to my brother really impacted my decision to go into to nursing to help people in need. What a rewarding feeling for my career choice to matter to someone's life every day. I can help people and make a difference.

But I will go out fighting for my child with every waking moment. He may have a shortened life, but it will be the best life ever. In 2009 we started a charity called Rally for Ryan. We have a lot of support from my parents and my brother. And we have the love from my husband's family and friends. This journey continues to evolve with the most wonderful people entering my son's life. Although my sisters have chosen to walk away and not be present in my son's life or my own, I will beat this in spite of it all. To walk away from a sick child is the ultimate betrayal of a family member. I thought living with a brother with Duchene would bond us together forever. I really thought my sisters who are mothers and could have just as easily had a baby with Duchenne would be champions of this cause, but they destroyed our family instead. My father just passed away a very sad man because of the way I was treated during this most painful, difficult event in my life. My son is 10 now and he once asked me why my sisters walked away from us? I said because they can.

I hope this story will honor all those who have passed away because of Duchenne.

We have come a long way from not having handicapped curbs and parking to now having the Americans with Disability Act, motorized wheelchairs, clinical trials and several ground breaking therapies on the horizon. I have come a long way from that little girl crying in the corner of my parent's bedroom to a champion for boys with Duchenne Muscular Dystrophy. My journey is not something I would have chosen but as my dad told me before he died, I know why you were chosen from our family because you will make a difference and you will never give up.

Epilogue

Please remember that our Duchenne Siblings are on the Duchenne journey for the rest of their lives. They will most likely be the ones making sure their brothers or sisters health care needs are being met when their parents are gone. And some will even have Duchenne children of their own. Their stories reveal the silent and not so silent pain, worry and fear they live with every day. They have a unique love and desire to protect their affected siblings as well as advocate for Duchenne in the most emotionally raw and forever way.

As you read their stories, you see how Duchenne forges them into the special adults they will become, filled with compassion and above all else, love. I also believe our Duchenne Siblings carry the torch for Duchenne eradication. We must not forget them.

Letter from the Editor

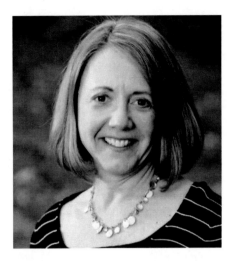

Editor, Lori Safford

It has been a privilege for me to edit the 20 stories in this book, *Don't Forget the Siblings*. Having two sons with Duchenne and a sibling myself, I know first-hand the difficulty of balancing the various needs of my three biological children, along with those of my step-son. Not only is it a challenge to meet the needs of a Duchenne Sibling, but simply deciphering what they are in the first place is a task in itself. This becomes even more impossible if they are teenagers!

This challenge was made considerably more difficult for me this past year when my husband unexpectedly passed away. Suddenly I was a single parent being pulled in a multitude of directions. I needed to figure out how to get Lydia home from volleyball or basketball practice when I was at swim therapy with Ben and Sam. And because of the boys' physical therapy appointments, I was only able to make about half of her games. What about when

Ben and Sam had a 3 hour power soccer practice and Lydia didn't want to attend? Should I leave my 13-year old at home alone or force her to come with us?

There are times when I have been up several nights in a row turning and caring for Ben and Sam and I am simply exhausted by the end of the week. The boys are tired as well and the three of us want to go to bed early on a Friday night, but Lydia wants to attend a church youth group activity which ends at 11:00pm. Do I make her sacrifice this activity so that the rest of us can get some well-needed rest? When I have attempted to do it all myself, I have ended up sick in bed or in the ER. Although my spirit is willing, my 50-year old body is simply weak. I have come to realize that I cannot be all things to all people…but this realization has not been easy to accept.

And those are just the social and logistical complications…what about the physical, psychological, emotional and spiritual ones? One thing I have learned is that we all grieve differently. Our Duchenne boys grieve the loss of their physical abilities differently than their parents or siblings do. With Duchenne, grief is cyclical; we are always grieving the loss of something: a dream, a physical ability, or a life.

Another thing I have come to realize is that although life is hard (and unfair), God is good. Through the unimaginable trials in life like the diagnosis of Duchenne and becoming a widow at 49, God has revealed His goodness, His provision and His strength. You have learned about some of the ways God has met the needs of other families and individuals as you have read the stories in this book.

Duchenne siblings grow up fast. They must deal with difficult issues and mature subjects at a very young age. It is almost like a piece of their childhood is lost; their innocence is somehow diminished. As I edited the stories in this book which were written by younger siblings (including the one written by my own daughter Lydia), I was genuinely amazed at the level of maturity, depth of character and strength of spirit revealed and I'm sure you will be too.

My prayer is that God has truly spoken to you through the pages of this book and that you will reach out to support, help and advocate for a Duchenne family near you.

Blessings,

Lori Safford

Lori Safford is mom to Ben, Sam and Lydia and step-mom to Kevin. After receiving her MA in Communications Management from Simmons College and working in the field of marketing and corporate communications for 17 years, she and her husband Mike made the decision for her to stay home full-time to care for their children. Ben and Sam were diagnosed with Duchenne shortly thereafter. Lydia also carries the genetic defect. Her husband Mike passed on in January of 2012 and the family has been adapting to its "new normal" ever since. Lori volunteers at her church and her children's Christian school and co-leads a Joni and Friends (www.joniandfriends.org) Moms Morning Out group for moms of kids with disabilities. She also serves on a human rights and behavioral review committee for a local NH agency that serves adults with developmental disabilities. In her spare time she trains and races in triathlons with the Gals for Cal (www.galsforcal.com) to raise money for Duchenne research. Her greatest joy is to watch her children serving others and glorifying the Lord in everything they do. She can be reached at lorisafford@comcast.net.

Who is Misty VanderWeele

I am Luke and Jenna's mom and Glen's wife. I have authored 4 Duchenne books. *In Your Face Duchenne Muscular Dystrophy All Pain All GLORY! Saving Our Sons One Story at a Time, Saving Our Sons and Daughter II*, and now this very book, *Don't Forget the Siblings*.

Although my son Luke age 21, passed on January 21, 2013 of complications from having Duchenne; only 14 days ago from the time I write this sentence, my commitment to helping others touched by Duchenne hasn't changed. If anything my resolve is even BIGGER and believe me -WAY STRONGER! The Duchenne story must be heard! Our Duchenne children deserve to live full long lives.

My mission is still the same. -To create an army of Duchenne parents, siblings, family and friends in what I call the Duchenne Movement. You can also find me in books, *Celebrating 365 Days of Gratitude and Adventures in Manifesting; Healing from Within*. It is time the world knows what Duchenne is. That is why I am committed to global Duchenne recognition. You can learn more about me at http://MistyVanderWeele.com. Be sure to check out my e-magazine, *THRIVE! --In the face of Duchenne Muscular Dystrophy* and the all new THRIVE Community while you are there.

Misty Gives Back

Duchenne Movement Book Affiliate Program

A portion of the proceeds of *Don't Forget the Siblings* will go to the co-authors who chose to become a Duchenne Movement affiliate. Such affiliates selling books will earn a commission based on books they sell. Such commissions can go towards expenses insurance won't cover, pay bills, give to their favorite Duchenne charity or to use toward something special for their Duchenne children. Herby any commissions earned by the affiliate/co-author will be spent at their discretion and are liable for any taxes due on such earned commissions. For more details about the Duchenne Movement Affiliate Program contact Misty VanderWeele at misty@mistyvanderweele.com.

Heart Shaped Rocks

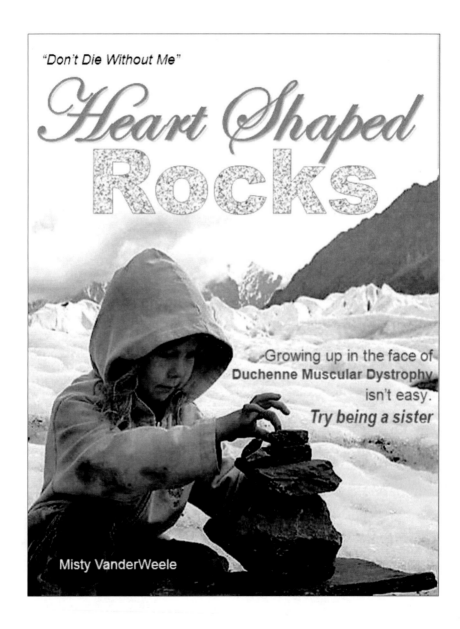

"Don't Die Without Me"

Heart Shaped Rocks

Growing up in the face of Duchenne Muscular Dystrophy isn't easy.
Try being a sister

Misty VanderWeele

♥

Heart Shaped Rocks is a story in progress. It is my daughter Jenna's story, a living story which unfolds little by little every day. You see, Jenna, like tens of thousands of other siblings, has spent her first 13 years on this planet knowing that her brother could die at any moment from complications of Duchenne Muscular Dystrophy, when suddenly he did.

(Duchenne Muscular Dystrophy or simply Duchenne or DMD as it is commonly referred to, is most common form of muscular dystrophy. It is a muscle wasting disease which mainly affects boys although girls can be diagnosed with it too. Its victims like my son Luke, are born seemingly healthy but as time goes on and the disease progresses, the body's muscles get thinner and weaker rending the child unable to walk. By the age of 10 or 12 a Duchenne child must use an electric wheelchair for mobility. A manual wheelchair isn't practical since he is usually too weak to propel himself. At the same time Duchenne takes away lower body strength, it starts affecting upper body strength, eventually destroying the heart and lungs which results in premature death in young adulthood, usually by the late teens or mid-twenties.

When Jenna was born her brother, Luke, was able to hold and feed her. In her toddler years she rode on the back of his electric wheelchair. By the time she was in elementary school, Luke was not able to lift his arms to hug her or even give her a brotherly slug in the arm. Although Jenna's story of life as a Duchenne sibling is heart breaking, I want you to know that like my first book, *In Your Face Duchenne Muscular Dystrophy, All Pain...All GLORY!,* this book is about making the very most out of what life throws at you while looking for those synchronistic signs and Aha moments that teach you that life is meant to be lived on purpose. This time, instead of telling the story of my son's battle with DMD, my intention is to honor my daughter's life as she watches how much Duchenne takes from her brother,

♥

while at the same time benefiting from all that it gives in terms of passion, maturity and strength of character.

As her mother, it's an honor to witness the transformation of a young girl into the young woman Jenna is becoming. She has so much to offer this world. Just wait until you read how on purpose and full of love for life Jenna is and how Duchenne has molded her. Living in the face of uncertainty has helped her develop into a young lady submerged in love for life, compassion, and the example of living grace. She gives her heart gently but full on. I am sure you'll fall in love with her one heart shaped rock at a time.

Heart Shaped Rocks (HSR) is divided into two different sections beginning with the news of my pregnancy with Jenna all the way to the present day with Jenna now being 13 years old. HSR details her journey as the progression of Duchenne ravages her brother's body and then takes his life. But first let me give you some background with which to lay out her story.

As a Duchenne carrier, I have a 50% chance of having a child born with Duchenne. And as I mentioned earlier, Duchenne mostly affects boys but girls can have it too (although that's very rare). So when my son was diagnosed back in 1995, I had decided there would be no more children for me. At that time I had just started a relationship with my now husband Glen and we decided that having one child would be enough for both of us. Besides, I knew what was to come in the future and I wasn't too sure I wanted to put this kind of grief into another person's life, let alone another child. However, life had a surprise in store for me.

That surprise being Jenna.

Currently, I live with my daughter, Jenna, and my husbands, Glen on our family's vegetable farm here in Alaska. Most people don't

♥

know but Alaska got started with agriculture back in 1935 through President Roosevelt's resettlement program. All though many farms are not in operation anymore, there are a handful of farmers left. Some of us are lobbying for Alaska to be a self-sustainable state. We live in a vast valley surrounded by mountains and glaciers. Our home in particular has an incredible view and numerous fields to roam, which we enjoy frequently. It's an incredible place to raise a family and grow a happy life. It's one of many things I am in awe of; I feel deeply grateful to get to live here and I embrace all that this home-spun family-farm lifestyle has to offer.

So what does heart shaped rocks have to do with living in the face of Duchenne? Well, you will learn just that as you continue to turn the pages of this book.

Chapter One, The heart of the matter

God wouldn't give me more than I could handle, right?

I used to have this idea that my son being dealt the hand of Duchenne was the end of all my troubles or at least that no new ones would appear. I believed that somehow I would get through this tragedy, help a bunch of other people in the process and then get on with life. Yes, it would hurt like hell but other parents had learned to go on after the death of a child. I figured I'd find a way to survive one way or another. For a while I also bought into the "there's nothing we can do so go home and enjoy your son while you still have him" mentality hook, line and sinker.

The *God wouldn't give me more that I could handle* saying was almost my mantra. I had absolutely no idea that once you start on the Duchenne journey, you are on the journey for life. Let's just say I didn't get the memo.

"You're pregnant".

♥

WHAT? This question screamed in my mind. I knew I hadn't been feeling well, but pregnant? No way is this happening. What was I going to tell Glen? We weren't even married yet. I knew that he hadn't wanted any children of his own; he had told me so, just like so many other guys have said. Luke was newly diagnosed with an incurable disease, and worse, this baby could have Duchenne too! I was just sick inside from this news. My friend who was with me at the time later told me I looked like I had just seen a ghost.

All I knew at that moment was that I would keep this baby no matter what. I took the long way home to absorb this new change in my life before springing the news on Glen. I was pretty sure Luke, who was 7 at the time, would be okay with the news, probably even excited. I also knew I had to be certain in my heart what I was going to do no matter what Glen decided.

If you read my first book, *In Your Face*, you know that Glen chose us, knowing that Luke had Duchenne, knowing there was a possibility the new baby would have Duchenne and all. We got married and committed to create the best life possible for our family. Luke was the ring bearer and both my boys wore mud flaps (what Glen told Luke the tales of their tuxedoes were).

Little Bird

After the initial shock of actually being pregnant wore off, I had this internal "knowing" the baby I was carrying was a girl. For obvious reasons besides already having a boy, I knew I needed this baby to be a girl. I wasn't so sure I could handle another blow. Her name was already Jenna, which means little bird. I was about 7 months along and even with all the previous ultra sounds, we couldn't tell the sex of the baby. My anxiety was high as I worried that my gut feelings might be wrong. I kept second guessing myself until one spring morning. I had been up

♥

all night with worry the night before. I had asked God to give me a sign if I was right about this baby being a girl. I got my answer.

I was getting ready to leave for my last ultrasound after working in our greenhouse that day. And up in the tree was this lone "little bird" singing its heart out. I cried all the way to the ultrasound appointment and when the doctor asked me if I knew the sex of the baby. I said, "She's a girl."

"Are you okay?"

Jenna was born on a sunny July morning. I immediately fell in love with her as she nursed and gazed into my eyes for the very first time. She was the most beautiful baby I'd ever seen. She was an angel. When all of a sudden up high on the left side of my body, in the high lung upper throat area was this intense pain that had me very uncomfortable. I felt like I had swallowed something entirely too big. One nurse asked me if I was okay. I said yes but I have this horrible pain and I grabbed where the pain was coming from. They whisked Jenna away from me. Gave me a shot of blood thinners and had me hooked up to almost every machine they had. Come to find out I had a pulmonary embolism, which means I had a blood clot in my lungs. They were very worried the clot would travel either to my brain or my heart. Although I was scared, I had my baby girl, my wonderful husband, and an incredible son with an uncertain future who needed me.

I had found a life I had never dreamed of and I wasn't going anywhere!

♥

Cheerio O's

We brought her home in a white eyelet lace baby bonnet. Over
the next month of newborn ness Jenna would make these O's
with her mouth as she looked around. She was often referred to
as, pumpkin, turnip and pickle as each of us had our own
vegetable names for her. She was the highlight of our lives. She
was our "little sprout." Her first Halloween we dressed her up as
a baby leopard, black nose and all. Then the first Christmas came.
We were totally enamored with her.

Whirl Wind

Great Grandma Mary from Texas called Jenna a little "Whirl
Wind" as Jenna ran through the house never missing a beat. And
her Great Oma on Glen's side would marvel over how
determined she was to learn new things. However I was starting
to notice the not so fun trait of her being overly sensitive and
whiney over very small things. This forced me to change my
parenting style since she'd thrown a fit from the pressure of
wanting to do good, but also not wanting to do what was
expected or being asked. On one hand I knew being a sensitive
person is a gift but on the other hand I worried about how we
were going to handle it as she got older.

Furniture to Furniture

As most babies do before they start to walk, Jenna found comfort
and more freedom going from one piece of furniture to another.
She was thrilled to be standing on her own and taking her first
steps. This is also when the progression of her brother's disease
was becoming more apparent. Luke was 8 years old and he

♥

reverted back to the comfort and safety of walking by going from one piece of furniture to the next. As Jenna started walking, her brother was taking his last steps. We knew the electric wheelchair wasn't too far ahead.

Brotherly Love

Luke was proud of Jenna; he loved her and continually showed his affection. There wasn't too much jealously on his part. Maybe it was all the years between them. But none-the-less, he felt very protective of her. I'd take him to her doctor's appointments with me. He would watch them like a hawk just waiting for them to mess up. Nobody was going to hurt his baby sister!

Road Kill

The Toddler years and Luke's first wheelchair found Jenna wanting to be a part of Luke's every waking moment. She loved riding on the back of his wheelchair and taking something Luke was using or playing with and running away. She knew Luke couldn't catch her. She would squeal and run. Luke would get fed up and tell her she was going to be "road kill." In no way was Luke ever going to hurt her. He was always fearful of running over her or hurting her in any way. But they were still siblings and kids will be kids.

Shared Custody

Luke's dad would come and pick him up for his two weeks every month. When Jenna was a baby she would cry and cry as she watched her brother leave. As his disease progressed the two

♥

weeks would turn into a time of doing things that her brother just couldn't physically do. It was also a time for resting up until he came home again. This was a time for her to be just Jenna.

Heart Shaped Rocks **Available Summer 2013**

♥

Other Duchenne Books Authored & Created By Misty VanderWeele

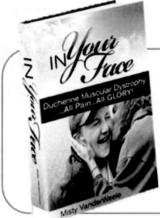

"*A beacon of light for others with the same challenges*" ~Patti B

A living memoir of mothers journey with sons life threatening disease, **Duchenne Muscular Dystrophy...**

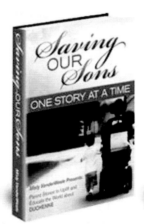

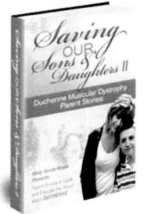

Over 80 combined personal stories to educate and uplift with world about **Duchenne Muscular Dystrophy...**

MistyVanderWeele.com

♥

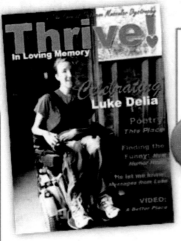

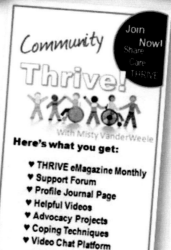
♥